Illustrated Manual of
NEUROLOGIC DIAGNOSIS

Illustrated Manual of
NEUROLOGIC DIAGNOSIS

R. DOUGLAS COLLINS, M.D., CAPTAIN, USAF, MC

*7505th USAF Hospital, R.A.F. Burderop, Wiltshire, England;
former special trainee for the National Institute of Neurological
Diseases and Blindness, Jefferson Medical College Hospital,
Philadelphia*

With a Foreword by RUDOLPH JAEGER, M.D.
*Professor and Chief, Department of Neurological Surgery,
Jefferson Medical College and Hospital, Philadelphia*

97 Illustrations of
Neurologic Diseases

J. B. LIPPINCOTT COMPANY
Philadelphia   •   Toronto

Distributed in Great Britain by
Pitman Medical Publishing Co., Limited, London

Library of Congress Catalog Card No. 62-8094

Printed in the United States of America

798

FOREWORD

A clear understanding of the numerous disorders of the nervous system is difficult to achieve, even though one is fairly well informed concerning anatomy, physiology and pathology, because of a wide gap both in visual retention and in translation from well-known facts to the essential knowledge for clinical interpretation. A feeling of frustration, which breeds disinterest, continues to prevent many physicians and medical students from attaining a practical working knowledge of the vast number of diseases that disturb the huge initiating and co-ordinating systems of the neuron complex that we call the nervous system. Any attempt to clear the fog from this cobweblike intermingling maze of tiny strands, which in fact has well-established orderly arrangements, is to be encouraged, commended and welcomed eagerly.

Busy, fatigued or even bright minds have had a tendency to relegate the study of nervous disorders to the background in favor of more easily understood, yet often less common or less important, afflictions of mankind. However, the fact remains that most physicians are forced to make fundamental decisions in neurology in caring for the sick.

In recent years determined efforts have been made to fill in the large gap between the fundamental, cold anatomic relations of the nervous system and its truly functional possibilities in clinical interpretation under normal conditions and in the presence of disease. This must be accomplished without robbing the student and the physician of valuable time needed for accumulating and perfecting knowledge and skill in the practical matters of other specialties. Few can afford to give up years, or even months, to the exclusive study of neurology; nor is it profitable in the long run for physicians concerned primarily with other branches of medicine to do this. Rather, it is better that one develop a continuing study technic whereby needed practical information can be obtained and applied as the occasion demands and the candidate for professional advancement grows in experience, skill and wisdom.

This book presents a much-needed and unique approach to the recognition, the illumination and the clarification of neuroanatomic and neurophysiologic facts as they are applied to clinical neurologic problems. A three-dimensional color-contrast display simplifies and intensifies the retained visual impression for instantaneous recall of needed combinations of facts to formulate a composite picture of the true identity of each well-known clinical syndrome. The brief yet clearly arranged outline of basic neurologic principles and symptomatology supplies the orientation required in attempting a systematic approach to the presenting problem. This, I think, is of the utmost importance to the beginner in neurology, as well as to the well-grounded practitioner who is desirous of retaining an active interest in all medical problems.

I believe that this book will prove to be of inestimable value in contributing to a more widespread practical knowledge of and interest in the neurologic sciences.

RUDOLPH JAEGER, M.D.

PREFACE

This book is not a substitute for definitive texts on neurologic diseases. Rather, it embodies a simplified approach to understanding that, at the very least, should encourage the physician to suspect neurologic disease. Used carefully, it can lead him systematically to a differential diagnosis.

Practical neurology is not the mysterious, esoteric science that it may seem to be. The long hours spent on the study of neuroanatomy in the freshman year of medical school are not wasted; with proper application, an understanding of neuroanatomy can unveil much of the mystery of clinical neurology.

THE DISEASE, THE NEUROANATOMIC LESION, THE NEUROLOGIC SIGNS

Two well-planned neuroanatomic drawings become the background on which are portrayed 79 important neurologic diseases. The neurologic signs of each disease are symbolized by shading or speckling the tracts, the nuclei or the regions involved—a method used by von Economo as early as 1924 and applied in many standard neurologic texts. In neurology, a knowledge of the location of the lesion provides a basis for the interpretation and the recall of the major signs of each disease. Says Sir Francis Walshe:

> When all due consideration has been given to the non-anatomical factors in neurological diagnosis, it has to be admitted that the main clinical features of nervous disease, especially of its more chronic varieties, are chiefly determined by the localization of the disease process within the nervous system.

The explanation of this basic principle is simple. The neuron's reaction to injury is stereotyped. It either dies or suffers at least a temporary arrest of function. Consequently, in most cases, neurologic signs are due to *loss of function* (paralysis, blindness, anesthesia) of the diseased area or *release or reorganization of function* (tremors, spasticity) of another area that formerly was inhibited by the area now diseased.

THE NEUROLOGIC SIGN, THE NEUROANATOMIC LESION, THE DIFFERENTIAL DIAGNOSIS

The location of the lesion is also the "common denominator" of the neurologic sign and the differential diagnosis. A knowledge of *where the lesion is* establishes the differential of *what the lesion is*. This is because different disease processes affect different functioning components of the nervous system.

This fundamental principle is the basis of the approach to diagnosis and the diagnostic tables presented in this book. Neurologic examinations, neurologic signs and neurologic disorders are cross-indexed with neuro-anatomic structures. While most students of neurology have at their command a sizable body of neuroanatomic and neurophysiologic facts, many of these facts are isolated. The diagnostic tables organize and correlate these facts so that they can be applied usefully in clinical neurologic problems. Also, they can serve as a guide to the study of standard neurologic texts.

To present neurology in a brief, organized fashion to students and general practitioners, an attempt has been made to adhere to the following criteria:

1. The backbone of this material is generally accepted information. Elaborate discussion of controversial theories, rare neurologic disorders and unusual case reports are omitted.

2. In general, neuroanatomic structures with obscure or rare clinical application are excluded from the drawings.

3. Complete discussions of each disease are replaced by typical case reports emphasizing those features with broader clinical application.

4. Descriptions of special diagnostic procedures performed almost exclusively by the specialist are omitted.

5. Treatment is summarized briefly by listing the "treatable disorders" and possible modes of therapy.

In simplifying any subject, particularly neurology, inevitably one is faced with the risk of being misleading, regardless of how accurate his material may be. However, it would seem to be a worth-while risk if it means teaching something otherwise regarded as impractical; if it means attracting to the field men who otherwise would be *alienated toward* it.

R. DOUGLAS COLLINS, Capt. USAF

ACKNOWLEDGMENTS

This work was inspired by Warren Blair and James Foley. Their continued interest in its progress and their assistance in its preparation have been most gratifying.

I am indebted to my teachers—Dr. Nathan Schlezinger, Dr. I. M. Tarlov and Dr. A. V. Jenson—for inculcating in me the basic principles of neurology, and to Dr. Walter Zerbe for many rich clinical experiences in neurologic diagnosis. The years spent with Dr. Paul Peck in learning the fundamentals of medical art allowed me to collaborate successfully with the talented Joseph Alemany in designing and preparing the illustrations that are the core of this manual. The supervision given by Dr. Remedios Rosales in placing the lesions in each disorder was of immense value.

I wish also to thank Dr. Raymond Joson, Dr. Howard Fields, Dr. William McLean and Dr. Nussret Mutlu, who offered much valuable criticism in the early stages of the work. I am obligated particularly to Dr. Clinton Pittman, who analyzed each proof critically and assisted me in numerous ways throughout the production of the book. Dr. Rudolph Jaeger's encouragement and assistance in the final stages of preparation were also of immeasurable help.

Of those many others who worked diligently at the task of preparation, I thank Mary Jane Croissant and Elaine Marghilano for their expert typing of the many revisions of the manuscript.

R. DOUGLAS COLLINS, M.D.

CONTENTS

PART I

xii   **Contents**

PART II

    Introduction to the Anatomic Profiles   47
    Section A: Lesions Below the Foramen Magnum
    A Summary of the Functional Anatomy of the Spinal Cord . .   48
        Master Plate I   49
    A. Degenerative and Demyelinating Diseases of the Cord
        Amyotrophic Lateral Sclerosis   50
        Friedreich's Ataxia   52
        Multiple Sclerosis   53
        Pernicious Anemia   56
        Progressive Muscular Atrophy   58
        Syringomyelia   59
        Werdnig-Hoffmann Disease   61
    B. Inflammatory Diseases of the Cord
        Epidural Abscess   62
        Herpes Zoster   63
        Infectious Polyneuritis   64
        Poliomyelitis   66
        Syphilitic Meningomyelitis   68
        Tabes Dorsalis   70
    C. Neoplasms of the Spinal Cord
        Extramedullary Spinal Cord Tumor   71
        Intramedullary Spinal Cord Tumor   75
        Cauda Equina Tumor   76
        Metastatic Carcinoma   77
    D. Vascular Diseases of the Cord
        Anterior Spinal Artery Occlusion   78
    E. Traumatic Disorders of the Spinal Cord
        Compression Fracture of Spine   79
    F. Diseases of the Spinal Column
        Cervical Spondylosis   80
        Osteoarthritis   81
        Ruptured Nucleus Pulposus   82
        Tuberculosis of the Spinal Column   85
    G. Diseases of the Peripheral Nerves
        Periarteritis Nodosa   86
        Diabetic Neuropathy   87
        Lead Neuropathy   88
        Nutritional Neuropathy   89
        Peroneal Muscular Atrophy   90

PART I

THE DIAGNOSTIC INTERPRETATION OF NEUROLOGIC SIGNS

Steps to a
Neurologic Diagnosis

The following outline summarizes the steps for arriving at a neurologic diagnosis with the use of the aids in this book:
1. The neurologic examination
2. Are the neurologic findings real or of localizing significance?
3. Where is the lesion responsible for the neurologic signs?
   A. What is the anatomic level of the lesion?
   B. Which tracts or nuclei are involved?
4. What is the lesion?
   A. Does the patient have a "treatable" disease?
      Does the patient have a space-taking lesion?
   B. Which diagnostic procedures confirm the diagnosis?

1. THE NEUROLOGIC EXAMINATION

The finer technics of the neurologic examination have been discussed repeatedly in many standard neurologic texts and handbooks; therefore, they are not elaborated upon here. Nevertheless, the routine neurologic examination has been illustrated on pages 8 to 13 to simplify the recall process. Once the routine examination is completed, the clinician may wish to substantiate his abnormal findings by further tests of the same tract, nucleus or region. These tests are indexed with the respective anatomic structures in Appendix A.

2. ARE THE NEUROLOGIC FINDINGS REAL OR OF LOCALIZING SIGNIFICANCE?

Special features of conversion hysteria are listed in Table 1. This disorder is a common cause of curious neurologic findings and often can be diagnosed by a careful examination. Frequently "abnormal" findings are due to associated metabolic disease (hyperthyroidism, drugs, etc.), increased intracranial pressure, or poor co-operation of the patient with low mentality, emotional instability, or subnormal levels of consciousness. Perhaps the findings are consistent with the patient's age. On the other hand, the patient's efforts to conceal his disabilities may yield a normal examination. These aspects of interpretation should not be neglected.

3

3. WHERE IS THE LESION RESPONSIBLE FOR THE NEUROLOGIC SIGNS?

The location of the lesion tells the surgeon where to operate. More important to the clinician, it is the key to a differential diagnosis. This process involves 2 phases: location on the longitudinal plane, i.e., the anatomic level; and location on the transverse plane, i.e., the tracts or the nuclei involved. Besides the tables, the two basic neuroanatomic drawings on pages 49 and 99 will assist the reader in this task. Each portrays longitudinal and transverse views of the nervous system.

What is the Anatomic Level of the Lesion?

For proper application of the diagnostic tables in this book, first it must be determined whether the lesion is above or below the foramen magnum. As a rule, if there are no cranial nerve signs, no papilledema, no nystagmus, no mental or speech changes and no seizure disorders, the lesion is below the foramen magnum. However, there are exceptions; for example, parasagittal lesions, early cerebellar lesions. Above the foramen magnum the lesion can be localized further to respective levels of the brain stem (medulla, pons, etc., Table 3) if there are cranial nerve signs (excluding supranuclear palsies). It can be localized to the cerebrum if there are overt mental or seizure disorders (excluding petit mal).

Generally, the lesion in neurologic disorders causes a "clinical level" corresponding to the anatomic level of the lesion. Again a notable exception to this principle occurs in lesions anywhere along the "axis" of the cerebellar system. Table 2 and the figures on pages 16 to 19 correlate the clinical and the anatomic levels in various lesions of the sensory and the motor pathways.* Signs explainable by a lesion at one level arouse suspicion of space-taking lesions (neoplasm, hematoma, abscess, etc.), the most urgent conditions in the differential diagnosis (see p. 6). If the findings will not fit a lesion at one level, a disease characterized by multiple lesions—for example, multiple sclerosis, neurosyphilis—should perhaps be considered.†

Which Tracts or Nuclei Are Involved?

In Tables 4 and 5 the abnormal findings are categorized according to the tract, nucleus or the region destroyed. If the anatomic level is below the foramen magnum, Table 4 is applicable. If the anatomic level is above

---

* The fact that the posterior and the lateral columns cross in the upper cord and the low brain stem, while fibers that contribute to the spinothalamic tracts cross near their level of origin, should be kept in mind when studying the figures.

† Rarely multiple lesions are explained by two or more conditions, one of which may be a space-taking lesion.

the foramen magnum, Table 5 is applicable. As the initial step, the tracts, the nuclei or the regions that best explain the neurologic signs in each case are selected. Then, a differential diagnosis of the principal diseases involving each tract, nucleus or region can be found in Table 6 (below the foramen magnum) or Table 7 (above the foramen magnum).

By locating the lesion on the two master illustrations (pp. 49 & 99), a comparison can be made with the lesions on the plates of each disease in the differential. As a further aid to diagnosis, case reports summarizing the most typical clinical features of each disorder accompany each plate. The following clinical case illustrates the steps taken in diagnosis to this point:

A 39-year-old white female complained of difficulty in walking and numbness and tingling in all 4 extremities for the past 6 months. Examination revealed increased patellar and Achilles reflexes, bilateral Babinski signs, loss of position and vibratory sense in both lower extremities, and a spastic-ataxic gait.

As there are no cranial nerve signs, papilledema, etc., in this case, a lesion would be suspected below the foramen magnum. The "Clinical Key to Involvement Below the Foramen Magnum," Table 4, indicates that involvement of the posterior and the lateral columns can cause these signs. Appendix A suggests that checking the patient further for graphesthesia, two-point sensibility, ankle clonus, etc., would confirm the signs of posterior and lateral column disease. In Table 6 and the color plates it is found that a differential diagnosis of posterior and lateral column destruction includes pernicious anemia, cord tumor, Friedreich's ataxia, multiple sclerosis, etc.

After repeated application of this method, means of shortening the process may come to mind. For instance, as indicated in Appendix B, lesions can be localized to a tract, a nucleus or a region with the knowledge of one neurologic finding; for example, Babinski sign. Other signs, however, can signify only involvement of a pathway or a system of two or more tracts and nuclei; for example, paralysis or anesthesia. Appendix C, which groups the disease into those with exclusively motor signs, those with exclusively sensory signs, or those with combined motor and sensory signs, provides another means of accelerating the process. For example, if the patient's signs are exclusively motor, most of the differential list can be arrived at with the use of the list in Group 1.

4. WHAT IS THE LESION?

By now one point should be clear. Knowing *where the lesion is* establishes a differential of *what the lesion is*. Some of the differential lists may overwhelm the reader at first glance. However, on closer inspection, he will note that the lists are classified according to the various etiologies (degenerative, inflammatory, neoplastic, etc.). In this way, the diseases can be correlated more efficiently with the historical findings (discussed below).

The understanding of neuroanatomy that leads to the differential can serve further in narrowing it. Obviously, if the signs indicate that two or more tracts or nuclei are involved, only those diseases that are classified mutually would be considered in the differential. Moreover, the diseases that invariably involve a tract, a nucleus or a region not suggested by the signs can be excluded. For instance, syringomyelia could be eliminated in the case given above because *almost consistently it involves* the ventral commissure.

The differential diagnosis of cranial nerve lesions can be reduced considerably if there are associated long-tract signs; i.e., to those conditions affecting the nerve or nucleus in the brain stem.

Diseases that characteristically cause symmetric lesions (spinocerebellar degeneration, pernicious anemia, nutritional neuropathy, muscular dystrophy, etc.) probably can be eliminated from the differential if there is exclusive unilateral involvement.

On the other hand, two diseases that cannot be eliminated anatomically —multiple sclerosis and neurosyphilis—must be included in practically every differential, because they may involve any part of the nervous system.

DOES THE PATIENT HAVE A "TREATABLE" DISEASE?*

To be practical, those diseases for which there is valuable therapy, Table 10, ought to be excluded from the differential first. In the diagnostic tables there is an asterisk beside each of these. The clinician who makes a "snap" diagnosis will want to be certain that he has not overlooked a "treatable" disease that also would explain his findings. He will find a differential of these conditions on each color plate.

Does the Patient Have a Space-Taking Lesion?

Of the "treatable" diseases and, thus, of all diseases in the differential, *the space-taking lesions deserve primary consideration.* Often, to overlook one of these is unnecessary disaster for the patient and the doctor's reputation. As suggested above, the clinician is alerted to these conditions if the findings are accounted for by a single-level lesion. Equally suspicious is unilateral involvement. Table 8 can be of great assistance in tracking down this possibility. Frequently, unequivocal exclusion of these disorders depends on special diagnostic procedures performed by a neurologic specialist (Table 9). Happily, the combination of early diagnosis and surgery often can save these patients from unnecessary disability or death.

* Whether a disease is treatable or not is to a certain extent a matter of opinion.

The Value of a Good History

While an extensive discussion of this topic is by-passed, this is not to belittle its time-proven value. Most commonly the final diagnosis is reached by reviewing the differential in the light of the findings from the history. Expensive laboratory tests can be circumvented safely by a good history. The following examples serve to emphasize its value:

The age of onset may establish the etiologic diagnosis. For instance, cerebrovascular diseases are rare below 20 years of age. Nevertheless, they may occur in association with sickle-cell anemia, subacute bacterial endocarditis, congenital heart disease or berry aneurysms.

The mode of onset also is significant. An acute onset would lead one to consider vascular, toxic or inflammatory disorders. A gradual onset would be more suggestive of neoplasms or degenerative diseases. Again, there are notable exceptions (and by now the reader should be thoroughly convinced that very little can be stated unequivocally in neurology). Generally, in tuberculosis and neurosyphilis the onset is insidious, while in metastatic carcinoma and glioblastoma multiforme it may be sudden.

The family history is extremely important in neurologic diagnosis. It may establish the diagnosis in spinocerebellar degeneration, muscular dystrophy, epilepsy and other disorders.

In the patient whose neurologic examination is negative, often the differential diagnosis depends on the history alone. However, it must be stressed that repeated neurologic examinations frequently are rewarding. Not a few neurologic disorders have exacerbations and remissions; for example, multiple sclerosis, myasthenia gravis. Three important symptoms that may occur without objective findings are headache, backache and convulsions. The differential diagnosis of these is discussed extensively in many contemporary texts.

WHICH DIAGNOSTIC PROCEDURES CONFIRM THE DIAGNOSIS?

Often, roentgenograms, laboratory and special diagnostic procedures are indispensable in establishing the exact diagnosis. Table 9 includes the most useful of these and important indications for their use.

By now it should be clear that establishing a diagnosis of neurologic disease is an orderly, logical gathering and interpretation of facts. The aids given in this book should make the process more understandable. The author hopes that the reader now possesses the ability to continue the study of neurology as he encounters the clinical entities in practice.

ILLUSTRATIONS OF THE ROUTINE NEUROLOGIC EXAMINATION

Mental Status:
  State of consciousness
  Orientation in time, space and
    person
  Memory of past and recent events
  Ability to count to and from 100
    by 1, 3, 7

Gait and Posture:
  Romberg

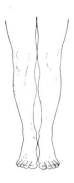

Gait

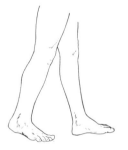

Ability to stand on each foot alone

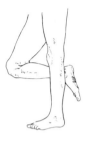

Ability to perform tandem gait

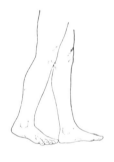

Ability to walk on heels or toes

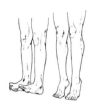

Skull:
Palpation for lumps and bumps

Auscultation for bruits

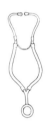

Visual acuity (II)

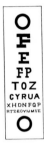

Pupil response (III)

Cranial Nerves:
Funduscopic examination (II)

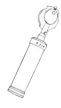

Visual fields (II)

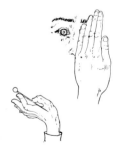

Extraocular movements (III, IV, VI), test for nystagmus (VIII)

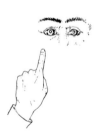

Palpebral fissures (III, cervical sympathetics)

Cranial Nerves—(Continued)
Corneal reflex (V, VII)

Facial muscle power (VII)
Jaw muscle power (V)

Sensation of face (V)

Palatal (X) and lingual (XII) power and bulk

Otoscopic examination (VIII)

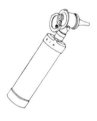

Trapezius power and bulk (XI)

Hearing (VIII)

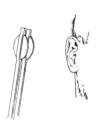

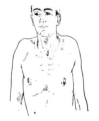

Upper Extremities:
  Motor System
    Co-ordination
      Finger-to-nose test

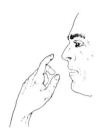

Patting test

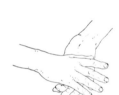

Power
  Hand grip

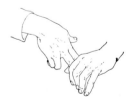

Abduction and adduction of fingers

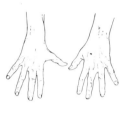

Extension and flexion of forearm and arm

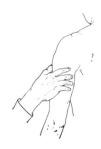

Muscle bulk and tone

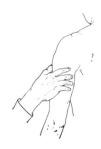

Upper Extremities—(*Continued*)
    Reflexes
        Triceps
        Biceps
        Brachioradialis

Pain

Stereognosis

        Hoffmann

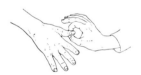

Lower Extremities:
    Motor System
        Co-ordination
            Heel-to-knee test

Sensory System
    Position sense

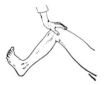

Vibratory sense

Power
    Flexion at knee

Lower Extremities—(Continued)
Extension at knee

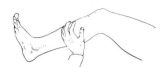

Plantar response

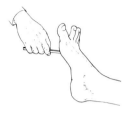

Flexion of toes and foot

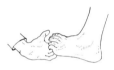

Sensory System
Position sense

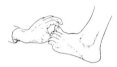

Extension of toes and foot

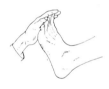

Vibratory sense

Muscle bulk and tone
Reflexes
   Patellar
   Achilles

Pain

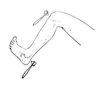

The Anatomic Location of the Lesion

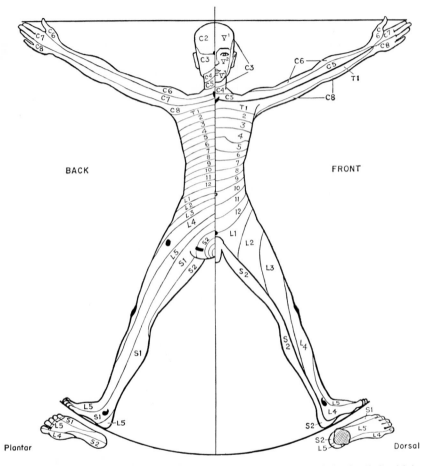

Dermatomes of human body from front (right side) and back (left side). After Keegan and Garret from Elliott, H. C.: Textbook of the Nervous System, ed. 2, Lippincott, Philadelphia.

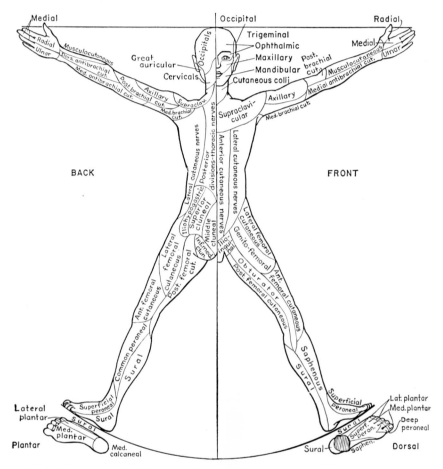

Dermal areas supplied by named nerves. Dermatomes and nerve areas do not coincide except where segmental structure still prevails. Elliott, H. C.: Textbook of the Nervous System, ed. 2, Lippincott, Philadelphia.

Correlation of the Sensory Level with the Anatomic Level of the Lesion

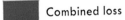 Combined loss

Analgesia

Loss of vibratory and position sense

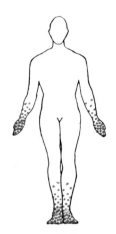

Multiple lesions of peripheral nerves (peripheral neuritis)

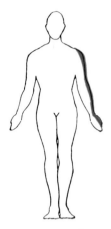

Cervical root lesion (C-6)

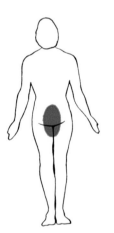

Cauda equina lesion

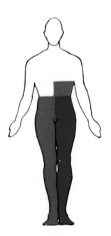

Left hemisection of thoracic cord (T-4)

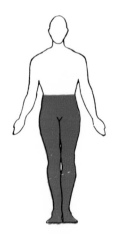

Complete transection of thoracic cord (T-7)

16

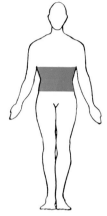

Early intramedullary
lesion of thoracic cord
(T-4 to T-9)

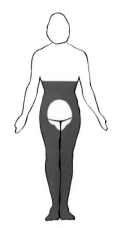

Advanced
intramedullary lesion
of thoracic cord
(T-4 to T-9)

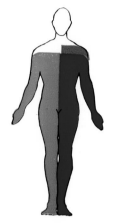

Left hemisection of
cervical cord (C-4)

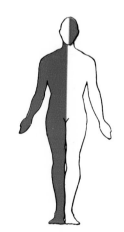

Left hemisection low in
brain stem

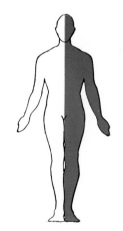

Right hemisection high in
brain stem

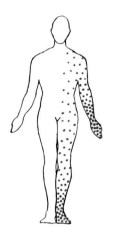

Right parietal lobe
lesion

Correlation of the Reflexes with the
Anatomic Level of the Lesion

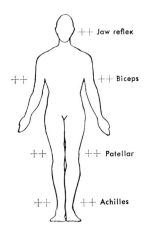

++ Jaw reflex

++   ++ Biceps

++   ++ Patellar

++   ++ Achilles

Normal reflex pattern

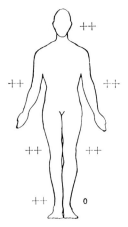

++

++   ++

++   ++

++   0

Lumbosacral root lesion
(L-5 to S-2)

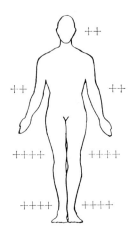

++

++   ++

++++   ++++

++++   ++++

Complete transection
of thoracic cord

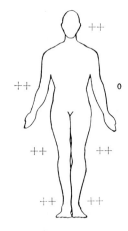

++

++   0

++   ++

++   ++

5th, 6th cervical root
lesion

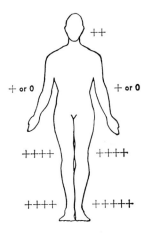

Complete transection
of low cervical cord
(C-5, C-6)

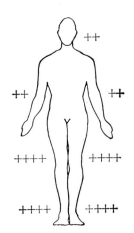

Parasagittal lesion

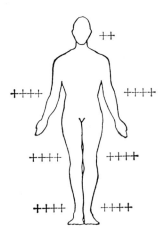

Complete transection at
foramen magnum or
low brain stem

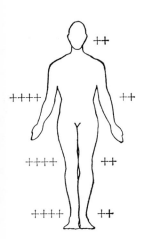

Left hemisection at
or above foramen
magnum

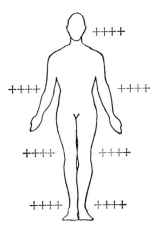

Complete transection
high in brain stem
(also a normal variant)

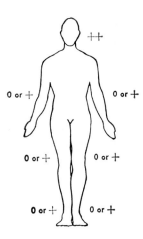

Multiple lesions of
peripheral nerves
(peripheral neuritis)

TABLE 1. EXAMPLES OF FINDINGS SUGGESTIVE OF HYSTERIA*

1. Mid-line anesthesia or analgesia

2. Inconstant pattern of sensory loss

3. Tuning-fork vibrations not felt on one side of skull

4. Complete loss of touch and pain without loss of temperature or position sense

5. Complete loss of position and vibratory sense in leg but ability to walk normally

6. Sensory loss not in conformity with an anatomic distribution

7. Complete blindness with pupils that react to light (exception: bilateral occipital lobe lesions, EEG helpful)

8. Tubular visual fields that remain the same size regardless of distance from examining chart

9. Paralyzed arm and hand not in the typical hemiplegic position (flexion of elbow, pronation of forearm, flexion of fingers only at interphalangeal joints)

10. Hemiplegia without greater distal paralysis

11. Tests for muscle power showing perhaps far greater disability than the performance in other tests would suggest (walking, co-ordination, etc.)

12. Objective parts of examination, such as optic fundi, reflexes normal

13. Hoover's sign: attempt by patient to raise paralyzed leg without thrusting normal leg downward

14. Adequate power in limbs in recumbent examination but complete inability to walk or stand (astasia-abasia)

15. Grand mal seizures without micturition, cyanosis, salivation or biting of tongue

---

* *Caution*: None of the above features is diagnostic of hysteria; nor can they exclude organic disease, as both may occur together.

TABLE 2. DETERMINATION OF ANATOMIC LEVEL OF LESION BY CLINICAL LEVEL OF PARALYSIS OR ANESTHESIA*

CLINICAL LEVEL OF INVOLVEMENT	PROBABLE ANATOMIC LEVEL OF SINGLE OR SPACE-TAKING LESION
Lower extremity	1. Below T-1 in cord (exception: parasagittal lesions) 2. Lumbosacral roots and plexus
Upper extremity alone	1. Cervical roots (e.g., cervical disk) 2. Brachial plexus (e.g., scalenus anticus syndrome) 3. Rarely peripheral cervical nerves (e.g., carpal tunnel syndrome, traumatic neuroma) 4. Early intramedullary cervical cord lesion
All four extremities	Cervical cord (exception: parasagittal lesions)
Head alone (cranial nerve signs)	1. Peripheral portion of cranial nerves (e.g., int. carotid aneurysm, pituitary adenoma, cerebellopontine angle tumor) 2. Early intramedullary involvement of brain stem (e.g., brain-stem glioma, pinealoma)
Head, upper and/or lower extremity	1. Cerebrum 2. Brain stem (e.g., advanced brain-stem glioma)

* This table deals only with single lesions. The location of multiple lesions is also possible in the peripheral nerves, at the myoneural junction and in muscle at any level.

TABLE 3. CLINICAL KEY TO THE LEVEL OF BRAIN-STEM INVOLVEMENT*

Medulla
1. Signs of involvement of one or more of the following cranial nerves: V, VIII, IX, X, XI, XII (see Clinical Key to Cranial Nerve Involvement)
2. Vertical and/or horizontal nystagmus
3. Hemiplegia, paraplegia, quadriplegia
4. Crossed hemianesthesia and/or hemianalgesia (may not be present above neck)
5. Dysmetria, dysdiadochokinesia, dyssynergia, intention tremor (usually unilateral)
6. Wide-base ataxic gait with falling to one side

Pons
1. Signs of involvement of one or more of cranial nerves V, VI, VII
2. Signs of upper motor neuron involvement of one or more of cranial nerves X, XI, XII
3. Paralysis of conjugate lateral gaze
4. Hemiplegia, paraplegia or quadriplegia
5. Crossed hemianesthesia and/or hemianalgesia
6. Internuclear ophthalmoplegia

Mid-brain
1. Signs of involvement of cranial nerves III or IV (infrequently Parinaud's syndrome)
2. Signs of upper motor neuron involvement of one or more of cranial nerves V, VII, X, XI, XII
3. Hemiplegia, paraplegia or quadriplegia
4. Hemianesthesia and/or hemianalgesia
5. Dysmetria, dysdiadochokinesia, dyssynergia, intention tremor usually unilateral
6. Head and posture tilt, wide-base ataxic gait

Diencephalon
1. Rarely visual field cuts
2. Signs of upper motor neuron involvement of one or more of cranial nerves V, VII, X, XI, XII
3. Hemiplegia (usually global) or quadriplegia
4. Hemianesthesia and/or hemianalgesia
5. Fleeting deep pains in face, arms and/or legs (thalamus)
6. Tremor, rigidity, chorea, athetosis

* One or more of the signs at each level may not be present in the individual case. Basically, the signs are some combination of cranial nerve and long-tract involvement, but either may occur alone.

TABLE 4. CLINICAL KEY TO THE INVOLVEMENT BELOW THE
FORAMEN MAGNUM*

Posterior Column

Numbness and tingling
Loss of vibratory sense
Loss of deep touch and position
  senses
Dysmetria

Loss of deep tendon reflexes
Ataxia accentuated by closing
  eyes
Romberg
Flaccid neurogenic bladder

Lateral Column

Weakness (diffuse but involves
  distal muscles more)
Loss of voluntary movement
Increased deep tendon reflexes
Ankle, patellar, wrist clonus
Babinski, Oppenheim, Chaddock,
  Hoffmann, Trömner

Loss of superficial abdominals
  and cremasteric reflexes
Muscle spasticity
Spastic gait
Spastic neurogenic bladder (can
  be flaccid in acute lesions)

Spinocerebellar Tracts

Usually no signs at all unless there
  is associated involvement of the

cerebellum (see Cerebellar
Hemispheres, p. 22)

Lateral Spinothalamic Tract

Contralateral changes

Loss of pain and temperature

Ventral Spinothalamic Tract

Contralateral changes

Loss of superficial touch (rarely)

Ventral Commissure

Bilateral changes

Loss of pain and temperature
senses

* Signs are homolateral unless otherwise specified. One or more signs under each
structure may be absent in individual cases. Losses may be total or partial.

TABLE 4—(*Continued*)

Sensory Root

Radicular pain (Lasègue's and Minor's signs)
Numbness and tingling
Loss of vibratory and position sense
Loss of touch, temperature, pain, in segmental fashion
Absent deep tendon reflexes without atrophy or reaction of degeneration
Flaccid muscles
Trophic changes
Broad-base ataxic gait accentuated by closing eyes
Flaccid neurogenic bladder if S 2, 3 or 4 is involved

Motor Horn or Root

Weakness (confined to individual muscles)
Loss of deep tendon reflexes
Muscular atrophy (more selective)
Fasciculations
Reaction of degeneration
Flaccid muscles
Loss of anal reflex and flaccid neurogenic bladder if S 2, 3 or 4 is involved
No pathologic reflexes
Vasomotor changes (if lateral horn is involved)

Peripheral Nerve

Weakness, paresthesia, pain
Tenderness of nerves and muscles
Nonsegmental combined sensory loss (e.g., glove and stocking)
Loss of vibratory and position sense
Absent deep tendon reflexes
Muscular atrophy
Fibrillations and reaction of degeneration
Trophic and vasomotor changes
Steppage gait

Sympathetic Ganglion

Horner's syndrome
Anhidrosis
Hypertension
Vasomotor changes (dermographia)

Muscles

Weakness (often proximal more than distal)
Atrophy (but occasional "hypertrophy")
No fasciculations or reaction of degeneration
Deep tendon reflexes retained until late, but diminished
Waddling gait

TABLE 5. CLINICAL KEY TO INVOLVEMENT ABOVE THE
FORAMEN MAGNUM

SECTION A: Major Tracts of Brain Stem*

Pyramidal Tract

Upper motor neuron involvement of one or more cranial nerves V, VII, X, XI, XII

Hemiplegia, quadriplegia

Babinski, Oppenheim, Chaddock, Hoffmann

Loss of superficial abdominals and cremasteric reflexes

Muscle spasticity

Spastic gait

Spastic neurogenic bladder

Medial Lemniscus

Numbness and tingling

Loss of vibratory sense

Loss of deep touch and position senses

Dysmetria

Ataxia accentuated by closing eyes

Romberg

Restiform Body or Brachium Conjunctivum

Homolateral changes

In-co-ordinated movements of extremities

Dysdiadochokinesia

Dyssynergia

Dysmetria often with intention tremor

Hypotonia

Decreased deep tendon reflexes (rarely)

Head tilt and posturing (occasionally)

Reeling, broad-base gait

Spinothalamic Tracts

Loss of pain and temperature

Loss of superficial touch (rarely)

SECTION B: Cerebrum, Extrapyramidal System, Cerebellum*

Frontal Lobe

Headache, focal, jacksonian or generalized motor seizures

Expressive aphasia

Confusion

Disorientation in time, space and person

Motor apraxia

Witzelsucht syndrome (excessive

jocularity; response to questions with silly answers)

Hemiplegia or monoplegia (usually with central facial palsy and often palatal or lingual weakness)

Grasp, after-grasp and sucking reflexes

---

* Signs are contralateral unless specified otherwise. One or more signs may be absent in any individual case. Losses may be total or partial.

Parietal Lobe

Headache

Jacksonian sensory seizures

Loss of vibratory and position sense

Graphanesthesia

Loss of two-point sensibility

Astereognosis

Temporal Lobe

Headache

Uncinate fits (unusual tastes, smells, hallucinations, déjà vu [already seen], psychomotor activity)

Auditory perceptive aphasia

Homonymous hemianopsia or quadranopsia

Occipital Lobe

Visual auras and seizures (flashes of light, blindness)

Homonymous hemianopsia, fre-

quently with macular sparing or incongruity

Parieto-occipital Junction

Visual perceptive aphasia

Nominal aphasia

Gerstmann's syndrome:

  Unable to differentiate right from left

Difficulty in performing simple arithmetic

Difficulty in differentiating one finger from another

Extrapyramidal System

Emotional instability (e.g., uncontrollable outbursts of laughter)

Masked faces

Myerson's eye signs

Monotonous speech

Fixed head and trunk

Muscular rigidity (cogwheel or plastic)

Involuntary tremor at rest (but disappearing during sleep)

Athetosis

Chorea

Hemiballism

Propulsion and retropulsion

Grotesque, clownish or short-step gait

Cerebellar Hemispheres

Homolateral changes

Syllabic or staccato speech

Nystagmus

In-co-ordinated movements of extremities

Dysdiadochokinesia

Dyssynergia

Dysmetria

Intention tremors

Hypotonia

Decreased deep tendon reflexes

Head tilt and posturing (occasionally)

Reeling, broad-base gait

Vermis of Cerebellum

Rocking forward and backward in Romberg position

Trunk ataxia

TABLE 5—(*Continued*)

SECTION C: Cranial Nerves*

I. *Olfactory Nerve*
   Loss of sense of smell

II. *Optic Nerve*
   Papilledema
   Papillitis
   Atrophy (primary and secondary)
   Central and paracentral scotomata
   Peripheral constriction of visual fields
   Sector field cuts (occasionally)
   Loss of visual acuity
   Optic Chiasma
   Bitemporal hemianopsia or quadranopsia
   Altitudinopsia (usually bilateral)
   Optic atrophy
   Paracentral scotomata (rarely)
   Optic Tract
   Contralateral homonymous hemianopsia (almost always without
      macular sparing)
   Wernicke's hemianopic pupillary response
   Optic Radiations
   Contralateral homonymous hemianopsia
   Quadranopsia (unilateral or bilateral)
   Occipital Lobe
   Contralateral homonymous hemianopsia (often with macular spar-
      ing)

III. *Oculomotor Nerve*
   Diplopia
   Lateral deviation of eye (exotropia)
   Paralysis of medial gaze
   Paralysis of upward gaze
   Paralysis of downward gaze
   Inability to elevate eye when turned medially
   Dilated fixed pupil (does not react to light accommodation or con-
      sensual stimulation)
   Loss of visual acuity
   Ptosis

* One or more signs may be absent in any individual case. Signs are homolateral
unless specified otherwise. Losses may be total or partial.

IV. *Trochlear Nerve*
    Diplopia
    Inability to depress eye when turned medially
    Head tilt away from side of paralysis
    Contralateral signs if lesion is nuclear

V. *Trigeminal Nerve*
    Sharp lancinating episodic neuralgia
    Nerve tenderness at areas of emergence of divisions of nerve
    Trigger zones of pain
    Loss of sensation to all modalities over forehead to bregma, over
        face excluding angle of jaw
    Loss of sensation to all modalities in oral cavity except taste
    Loss of corneal reflex
    Weak bite
    Loss of jaw jerk (increased in supranuclear palsy)

VI. *Abducens Nerve*
    Diplopia
    Medial deviation of eye (esotropia)
    Paralysis of lateral gaze

VII. *Facial Nerve*
    Ironing out of nasolabial fold
    Widened palpebral fissure (peripheral paralysis only*)
    Loss of ability to elevate eyebrows (peripheral paralysis only)
    Loss of ability to close eye tightly (peripheral paralysis only)
    Loss of ability to show teeth and smile
    Loss of ability to whistle
    Bell's phenomena (peripheral paralysis only)
    Loss of taste on anterior two thirds of tongue
    Weak corneal reflex
    Fasciculations of facial muscles (peripheral paralysis only)
    Blepharospasm

VIII. *Cochlear Nerve*
    Loss of ability to hear wrist watch or whispered voice
    Rinne test yields a 1:2 ratio of BC:AC despite loss of hearing
    Weber test lateralizes to side opposite lesion
   Vestibular Nerve
    Horizontal nystagmus (slow component usually to side of lesion)
    Past-pointing (to side of lesion)
    Diminished response to caloric testing

* "Peripheral" here meaning all parts of lower motor neuron.

TABLE 5—(*Continued*)

IX. *Glossopharyngeal Nerve*
  Loss of sensation in oropharynx
  Loss of sensation on posterior one third of tongue
  Loss of gag reflex

X. *Vagus Nerve*
  Elevation of palate to side opposite the weakness
  Loss of gag reflex
  Paralysis of vocal cord
  Difficulty in swallowing
  Dysarthria

XI. *Spinal Accessory Nerve*
  Weakness in elevation of shoulder
  Weakness in turning head to opposite side
  Atrophy and fasciculations of trapezius and sternocleidomastoid
    (peripheral paralysis only)

XII. *Hypoglossus Nerve*
  Deviation of tongue to side of weakness
  Atrophy and fasciculations of tongue (peripheral paralysis only)

The Differential Diagnosis

In general, the following etiologic classification has been adhered to in the formulation of the tables:

1. Degenerative and Demyelinating Disorders
2. Inflammatory and Toxic Disorders
3. Neoplasms
4. Vascular Disorders
5. Traumatic Disorders
6. Diseases of the Spine or the Skull
7. Miscellaneous Conditions.

In the tables on the cranial nerves and the major tracts in the brain stem, these categories are not listed specifically. Only the more common disorders are listed; these tables are not to be regarded as complete.

TABLE 6. DIFFERENTIAL DIAGNOSIS OF LESIONS BELOW THE FORAMEN MAGNUM

Anatomic Classification

Etiologic Classification	Posterior Column	Lateral Column	Spinocerebellar Tracts	Spinothalamic Tracts	Ventral Commissure
Degenerative and demyelinating disorders	Friedreich's ataxia Multiple sclerosis *Pernicious anemia Syringomyelia (late)	Amyotrophic lateral sclerosis Friedreich's ataxia Multiple sclerosis *Pernicious anemia Syringomyelia (late)	Friedreich's ataxia Multiple sclerosis Syringomyelia (late)	Multiple sclerosis Syringomyelia	Syringomyelia
Inflammatory and toxic disorders	*Epidural abscess *Syphilitic meningomyelitis *Tabes dorsalis Transverse myelitis	*Syphilitic meningomyelitis Transverse myelitis Epidural abscess	*Syphilitic meningomyelitis Transverse myelitis	Transverse myelitis	*Syphilitic meningomyelitis Transverse myelitis
Neoplasms	Angiomas Gliomas *Meningioma *Neurofibroma Metastatic neoplasms	*Neoplasms (as listed under Posterior Column)	*Neoplasms (as listed under Posterior Column)	*Neoplasms (as listed under Posterior Column)	Intramedullary neoplasms (ependymoma, etc.)
Vascular disorders		Ant. spinal artery occlusion		Ant. spinal artery occlusion	Ant. spinal artery occlusion
Traumatic disorders	*Compression fracture Contusion	*Compression fracture Contusion	*Compression fracture Contusion	*Compression fracture Contusion	Contusion
Diseases of the spine	*Cervical spondylosis	*Cervical spondylosis *Ruptured nucleus pulposus *Tuberculosis of the spinal column			
Miscellaneous	Arachnoiditis	Arachnoiditis			

* Denotes the "treatable" disorders.
Note: To be included in the differential does not necessarily imply involvement or vice versa.

TABLE 6 (Continued)

Anatomic Classification

Etiologic Classification	Sensory Root	Motor Horn or Root	Peripheral Nerve	Myoneural Junction or Muscle
Degenerative and demyelinating disorders		Amyotrophic lateral sclerosis Peroneal muscular atrophy Progressive muscular atrophy Syringomyelia Werdnig-Hoffmann disease	Peroneal muscular atrophy	Muscular dystrophy Myotonia dystrophica
Inflammatory and toxic disorders	Herpes zoster Infectious polyneuritis *Tabes dorsalis	Infectious polyneuritis *Lead neuropathy Poliomyelitis Transverse myelitis	*Alcoholic neuritis Arsenical neuritis Collagen disorders Diabetic neuropathy Infectious polyneuritis *Lead neuropathy *Nutritional neuropathy Porphyria Sulfonamides	Dermatomyositis Fibromyositis Trichinosis
Neoplasms	*Meningiomas *Neurofibromas Metastatic neoplasms	*All neoplasms (as listed under Posterior Column)	*Neurofibromas	
Vascular disorders		Ant. spinal artery occlusion		
Traumatic disorders	*Compression fracture	*Compression fracture Contusion	Transection *Traumatic neuromas	
Diseases of the spine	*Ankylosing spondylitis *Cervical spondylosis Osteoarthritis *Ruptured nucleus pulposis *Spondylolisthesis *Tuberculosis of spine	Diseases of the spine (as listed under Sensory Root)		
Miscellaneous	Arachnoiditis	Arachnoiditis	*Scalenus anticus syndrome	*Familial periodic paralysis Myotonia congenita *Myasthenia gravis

TABLE 7. DIFFERENTIAL DIAGNOSIS OF LESIONS ABOVE THE FORAMEN MAGNUM

Section A: The Major Tracts in the Brain Stem and Their Connections

Tract	All Levels	Additional Diseases at Various Levels*			
		Medulla	Pons	Mid Brain	Diencephalon
Pyramidal tract (not including cortical portion)	Amyotrophic lateral sclerosis Multiple sclerosis *Neurosyphilis Encephalitides *Primary neoplasms Metastatic neoplasms Basilar artery occlusions, *aneurysms and insufficiency	*Foramen magnum tumors	Pontine glioma Millard-Gubler's syndrome	Pinealoma (advanced) Mid-brain glioma Weber's syndrome	Anterior choroidal artery occlusion Intracerebral hemorrhage Lenticulostriatal artery occlusion or hemorrhage
Medial lemniscus	Multiple sclerosis *Neurosyphilis *Primary neoplasms Metastatic neoplasms Basilar artery occlusion or *insufficiency	Syringobulbia (late) *Vertebral artery occlusion or insufficiency	Pontine glioma	(rarely involved here)	Thalamic syndrome (this tract terminates here)
Restiform body		Multiple sclerosis Syringobulbia *Cerebellopontine angle tumor Post. inf. cerebellar artery occlusion *Vertebral aneurysm *Platybasia			
Brachium conjunctivum			(rarely involved here)	Multiple sclerosis Mid-brain glioma Benedikt's syndrome Basilar artery occlusion	
Spinothalamic tracts	Multiple sclerosis Brain-stem gliomas Basilar artery occlusion or *insufficiency	Syringobulbia Post. inf. cerebellar artery occlusion	Pontine glioma	(rarely involved here)	Thalamic syndrome (these tracts terminate here)

* The differential at any level must include those conditions listed under All Levels.

Note: The major tracts in the brain stem and their connections infrequently are involved in the brain stem without cranial nerve involvement.

TABLE 7 (Continued)

Section B: The Cerebrum, the Cerebellum and the Extrapyramidal System

Anatomic Classification

Etiologic Classification	Cerebrum	Cerebellum	Extrapyramidal System
Degenerative or demyelinating disorders	Diffuse sclerosis Lipoidosis Multiple sclerosis Senile and presenile dementia	Multiple sclerosis Parenchymatous cerebellar degeneration Spinocerebellar degeneration	Dystonia musculorum deformans Huntington's chorea *Paralysis agitans *Wilson's disease
Inflammatory or toxic disorders	*Epidural abscess *General paresis Inflammatory and toxic encephalopathies Meningo-encephalitis *Parenchymal abscess *Tuberculoma	*Cerebellar abscess Toxic encephalopathy due to alcohol *bromides diphenylhydantoin	Encephalitides *Phenothiazine intoxication Sydenham's chorea
Neoplasm	*Angiomas *Gliomas *Meningiomas Metastatic neoplasm	*Astrocytomas *Medulloblastomas *Meningioma Metastatic neoplasm	*Gliomas

Vascular disorders	Arterial
	  *Aneurysms
	  *Embolisms
	  Hemorrhage
	  Thrombosis
	*(Special: internal carotid thrombosis)
	*Arteriovenous anomalies
	*Venous sinus thrombosis
		*Basilar artery occlusion or insufficiency
		Occlusion of superior cerebellar artery
			Thalamic syndrome

Traumatic disorders	Contusion *Depressed fracture *Epidural hematoma *Subdural hematoma	*Depressed fracture	
Miscellaneous disorders	Cerebral palsy Idiopathic epilepsy	Acute cerebellar ataxia in children	Choreo-athetosis of cerebral palsy Senile tremors

TABLE 7 (Continued)

Section C: The Cranial Nerves and Their Connections (from peripheral to central)

	I Olfactory Nerve	II Optic Nerve	III Oculomotor Nerve IV Trochlear Nerve
End organ, muscle or myoneural junction	Rhinitis	*Keratitis *Cataract *Glaucoma Macular degeneration Chorioretinitis Retinitis pigmentosa *Occlusion of ophthalmic artery *Temporal arteritis *Occlusion of int. carotid *Retinal vein thrombosis	Progressive ophthalmoplegia Congenital ophthalmoplegia Myotonia dystrophica *Exophthalmic goiter *Myasthenia gravis *Orbital cellulitis
Peripheral portion of nerve		Leber's optic atrophy Neuritis Alcohol Diabetes Multiple sclerosis Syphilis *Sphenoid sinusitis Optic nerve glioma *Sphenoid ridge meningioma *Sellar and suprasellar tumors *Cerebral aneurysms Orbital trauma Basilar arachnoiditis *Pseudotumor cerebri	Diabetic neuropathy *Sphenoid sinusitis *Tuberculous meningitis *Sellar and suprasellar tumors Extension of nasopharyngeal neoplasms *Sphenoid ridge meningiomas *Cerebral aneurysms *Thrombosis of cavernous sinus
Portion of nerve or nucleus in brain stem	*Olfactory groove and *sphenoid ridge tumors *Frontal lobe tumors Trauma to anterior fossa	(Lesions of the optic tracts and lateral geniculate bodies are rare)	Multiple sclerosis *Syphilis Encephalitides *Wernicke's encephalopathy Brain-stem glioma Weber's syndrome (does not involve IV)
Supranuclear connections		Diffuse sclerosis *Temporal and occipital lobe space-occupying lesions Occlusion of posterior cerebral artery	Pinealoma

TABLE 7 (Continued)

	V Trigeminal Nerve	VI Abducens Nerve	VII Facial Nerve	VIII Cochlear and Vestibular Nerves
End-organ, myoneural junction or muscle		See oculomotor nerve	Muscular dystrophy Myotonia dystrophica *Myasthenia gravis	*Otitis media Otosclerosis Acute labyrinthitis *Ménière's disease
Peripheral portion of nerve	*Orbital cellulitis *Gradenigo's syndrome *Tuberculous meningitis Herpes zoster *Sphenoid ridge meningioma *Cerebellopontine angle tumors Nasopharyngeal neoplasms *Cerebral aneurysms Skull fracture *Tic douloureux	Conditions listed under oculomotor nerve *Gradenigo's syndrome (petrositis) *Cerebellopontine angle tumor Increased intracranial pressure	*Otitis media and petrositis 'Tuberculous meningitis *Syphilitic pachymeningitis Infectious polyneuritis Herpes zoster (Ramsay-Hunt syndrome) *Cholesteatoma *Cerebellopontine angle tumor *Tumor of glomus jugular *Vertebral-basilar aneurysms Fracture of petrous bone *Bell's palsy	Streptomycin intoxication *Syphilitic pachymeningitis *Tuberculous meningitis *Cholesteatoma *Cerebellopontine angle tumor *Vertebral-basilar aneurysm Fracture of petrous bone Vestibular neuronitis
Portion of nerve or nucleus in brain stem	Amyotrophic lateral sclerosis Multiple sclerosis Syringobulbia Pontine glioma	Conditions listed under oculomotor nerve (except Weber's syndrome) *Cerebellar tumor or abscess Millard-Gubler's syndrome	Amyotrophic lateral sclerosis Poliomyelitis Pontine glioma Basilar artery occlusion Millard-Gubler's syndrome	Multiple sclerosis Syringobulbia Meningoencephalitis Pontine glioma Posterior inferior cerebellar artery occlusion
Supranuclear connections	Pseudobulbar palsy (see differential of pyramidal tract and cerebrum)		Pseudobulbar palsy	

TABLE 7 (Continued)

	IX Glossopharyn-geal Nerve	X Vagus Nerve	XI Spinal Accessory Nerve	XII Hypoglossus Nerve
Muscle or myoneural junction		Vocal cord *Syphilis *Tuberculosis *Neoplasms *Myasthenia gravis	Muscular dystrophy *Myasthenia gravis	
Peripheral portion of nerve	*Foramen magnum tumors *Jugular vein thrombosis Glossopharyngeal neuralgia *Platybasia	**Extracranial portion** Riedel's struma Mediastinitis Thyroid tumor Mediastinal neo-plasms Aortic aneurysms Mitral stenosis **Intracranial portion** *Syphilitic pachy-meningitis *Tuberculous meningitis *Foramen magnum tumor *Tumor of ganglion nodosa *Vertebral-basilar aneurysms and *insufficiency *Jugular vein thrombosis *Platybasia Skull fracture	*Foramen magnum tumors *Vertebral-basilar aneurysm *Dislocation of upper cervical vertebrae Trauma to neck *Platybasia	*Tuberculous meningitis *Foramen magnum tumors *Vertebral aneurysm *Jugular vein thrombosis *Platybasia
Portion of nerve or nucleus in brain stem	(Rarely affected here; but differential similar to X)	Amyotrophic lateral sclerosis Syringobulbia *Syphilis Encephalitides Poliomyelitis Ependymoma of IVth ventricle Posterior inferior cerebellar artery occlusion	Amyotrophic lateral sclerosis Syringobulbia Poliomyelitis	Amyotrophic lateral sclerosis Syringobulbia Poliomyelitis Ependymoma of IVth ventricle
Supranuclear connections		Pseudobulbar palsy	Pseudobulbar palsy	Pseudobulbar palsy

TABLE 8. INDICATIONS OF SPACE-TAKING LESIONS*

1. *Space-taking lesions at and above the foramen magnum*

   A. Persistent headache, not usually relieved by analgesics and occasionally accompanied by vomiting

   B. Progressive onset of symptoms

   C. History of recent infection, trauma or neoplasm elsewhere

   D. History of focal or generalized seizures

   E. Personality changes

   F. Slow onset of hemiplegia

   G. Papilledema, increased intracranial pressure, or both

   H. Visual field cuts

   I. Unilateral perceptive deafness

   J. Other unilateral cranial nerve palsies

2. *Space-taking lesions below the foramen magnum*

   A. Radicular pain

   B. Progressive onset of symptoms

   C. History of recent infection, trauma or other neoplasm

   D. Slowly progressive onset of paraplegia, monoplegia or hemiplegia

   E. Sensory level

   F. Unilateral or bilateral atrophy of muscles at level of lesion

   G. Bladder and rectal sphincter disturbances

---

* If the patient has any of these findings, hospitalization for thorough history, neurologic and laboratory examinations (Table 9) is in order.

TABLE 9. DIAGNOSTIC PROCEDURES

LABORATORY STUDIES	SOME IMPORTANT INDICATIONS
c. b. c., indices, gastric analysis, Schilling test	Pernicious anemia
Alkaline phosphatase	Metastatic carcinoma
2-hour postprandial blood sugar	Diabetic neuropathy
Blood potassium level	Familial periodic paralysis
Blood lead level	Lead encephalopathy and neuritis
Blood Wassermann	Neurosyphilis
Blood bromide level	Bromism
C.S.F.-pressure	Space-taking lesions, subarachnoid and cerebral hemorrhages
C.S.F.-red cell count	Subarachnoid, cerebral hemorrhages
C.S.F.-leukocyte count	Bacterial meningitis, cerebral abscess
C.S.F.-sugar and chloride	Bacterial meningitis
C.S.F.-protein	Space-taking lesions, infectious polyneuritis
C.S.F.-acid fast smear	Tuberculous meningitis
C.S.F.-India ink smear	Cryptococcal meningo-encephalitis
C.S.F.-Wassermann	Neurosyphilis
C.S.F.-colloidal gold	Neurosyphilis and multiple sclerosis
Protein-bound iodine, R.A.I. uptake	Pituitary adenoma or craniopharyngeoma
Glucose tolerance test	Pituitary adenoma or craniopharyngeoma
Serum electrolytes	Pituitary adenoma or craniopharyngeoma
17-ketosteroids	Pituitary adenoma or craniopharyngeoma
Intake and output	Pituitary adenoma or craniopharyngeoma
Urine barbiturates	Barbiturate intoxication
Urine copper	Wilson's disease
Urine porphobilinogen	Porphyria

TABLE 9—(*Continued*)

STUDIES BY SPECIALISTS IN ALLIED FIELDS	SOME IMPORTANT INDICATIONS
Visual fields	Chiasmal and occipitotemporal lobe tumors, differentiation of optic neuritis from papilledema
Ophthalmodynamometry	Carotid artery thrombosis
Audiogram	Cerebellopontine angle tumor or cholesteatoma
Caloric tests (vestibular function)	Cerebellopontine angle tumor or cholesteatoma
Laryngoscopy	Vagus nerve lesions
Psychometric testing	Space-occupying lesions of cerebrum and cortical atrophy of various causes
Cystometric testing (bladder function)	Cord tumor, many inflammatory and degenerative lesions of cord and brain stem
ROENTGENOGRAMS	
Skull series	Lesions at and above the foramen magnum
Orbits	Sphenoid ridge meningioma, optic nerve glioma, orbital tumors
Auditory meati	Cerebellopontine angle tumor
Sinuses and mastoids	Brain abscess, cholesteatoma
Spine (cervical, thoracic, lumbar)	Lesions below the foramen magnum
Long bones	Metastasis, lead poisoning
Tomography	Closer identity of many lesions observed on other roentgenograms
SPECIAL ROENTGENOGRAMS BY NEUROLOGISTS AND NEUROSURGEONS	
Pneumoencephalogram	Space-taking lesions above cord, cortical atrophy of various causes
Ventriculogram	Space-taking lesions with increased intracranial pressure
Myelogram	Space-taking lesions of cord

TABLE 9—(*Continued*)

SPECIAL ROENTGENOGRAMS— (*Continued*)	SOME IMPORTANT INDICATIONS
Arteriogram	Space-taking lesions of brain; identity of aneurysms, arteriovenous malformations, angiomas, vascular occlusions
ELECTRICAL TESTS	
Electrocardiogram	Cerebrovascular disease, syncope
Electroencephalogram	Idiopathic epilepsy, space-taking lesions of cerebrum, cortical atrophy, hysteria
Electromyography	Anterior horn cell damage, peripheral neuritis, muscular dystrophy
STIMULATION TESTS	
Tensilon test	Myasthenia gravis
Histamine test	Migraine, histamine cephalalgia
Carotid compression test	Carotid artery thrombosis
Carotid sinus massage	Carotid sinus syncope
Cocaine dilatation of pupil	Horner's syndrome
Mecholyl constriction of pupil	Adie's tonic pupil vs. Argyll Robertson pupil
SURGICAL DIAGNOSTIC PROCEDURES	
Subdural taps	Subdural hematoma in infants
Muscle biopsy	Muscular dystrophy, periarteritis nodosa, trichinosis
Brain biopsy	Cortical atrophy of various causes
Nerve blocks	Hysteria, somatic vs. visceral pain
Bone biopsy	Metastatic carcinoma, reticuloendothelioses
Bone-marrow study	Pernicious anemia, multiple myeloma

TABLE 10. THE "TREATABLE" NEUROLOGIC DISORDERS

1. SURGERY

A. Space-Taking Lesions
   a. **Abscesses: epidural, subdural, brain substance**
   b. **Aneurysms and A-V anomalies**
   c. **Cervical spondylosis**
   d. **Hematomas: epidural, subdural, brain substance**
   e. **Neoplasms** (consider radiotherapy)
   f. **Herniated disks**

B. Miscellaneous
   a. **Common carotid thrombosis**
   b. **Compression fracture**
   c. **Hydrocephalus**
   d. **Ménière's disease** (in persistent cases)
   e. **Parkinsonism** (in selected cases)
   f. **Peripheral nerve injury and traumatic neuromas**
   g. **Trigeminal neuralgia** (in persistent cases)

2. MEDICAL THERAPY

A. Nutritional Disorders
   a. **Nutritional and metabolic neuropathies (in beriberi, pellagra, diabetes, alcoholism):** thiamine, nicotinic acid, physiotherapy
   b. **Pernicious anemia:** vitamin B_{12}
   c. **Wernicke's encephalopathy:** thiamine

B. Inflammatory Disorders
   a. **Abscesses (epidural, subdural, or in the brain substance):** antibiotics and chemotherapy
   b. **Bacterial and fungal meningitis:** antibiotics and chemotherapy
   c. **Neurosyphilis:** penicillin, typhoid fever therapy
   d. **Sinus thrombosis:** antibiotics
   e. **Tuberculosis of meninges and spinal column:** streptomycin, P.A.S., isoniazid

(*Note:* It is not to be implied from this table that therapy of neurologic disorders is so simple as to be limited to a few pages. However, these are the most important treatable disorders. Exact doses are omitted purposely to stimulate further investigation of treatment. Treatment, whether it is surgical, medical or a combination of both, must be evaluated in each case. For further discussion Forster's *Modern Therapy in Neurology* is recommended.)

TABLE 10—(*Continued*)

2. MEDICAL THERAPY—(*Continued*)
   C. Toxic Disorders
     a. **Bromism:** withdrawal of drug, sodium chloride by infusion or orally
     b. **Lead neuritis and encephalopathy:** calcium versenate

   D. Vascular Disorders
     Thrombo-embolic and vasospastic cerebrovascular disorders: vasodilators, anticoagulants, physiotherapy

   E. Idiopathic Disorders
     a. **Bell's palsy:** ACTH, cortisone, physiotherapy
     b. **Epilepsy:** phenobarbital, diphenylhydantoin, Tridione, etc.
     c. **Infectious polyneuritis:** ACTH
     d. **Ménière's disease:** diet, Antivert, histamine desensitization
     e. **Migraine headaches:** ergotamine
     f. **Myasthenia gravis:** Prostigmin, Mestinon, Mytelase
     g. **Parkinsonism:** Cogentin, Artane, Kemadrin, physiotherapy and exercise
     h. **Ruptured disks, cervical spondylosis:** traction, muscular relaxants, physiotherapy
     i. **Trigeminal neuralgia:** Dilantin, Trilene inhalation
     j. **Wilson's disease:** copper-free diet, BAL

PART II

ANATOMIC PROFILES OF
NEUROLOGIC DISEASES

Introduction to the
Anatomic Profiles

The anatomic profiles presented in the following pages of this book symbolize the major signs and symptoms of neurologic disease. With them it has been possible to circumvent a wealth of written description of neurologic diseases. The author hopes that once the reader has become acquainted with these "exercises in applied anatomy and physiology," he will enjoy using the plates in localizing the lesions in all his clinical cases.

The first series of plates are those of lesions *below the foramen magnum*. As an aid in remembering the tracts and the nuclei here, a mnemonic device has been devised. A cross section of the cervical spinal cord can be made to resemble a "face" simply by delineating the ventral commissure in the form of a "mouth." This represents adequately almost any level of the cord and simplifies the learning and recall process.

The second series of plates portray diseases of the structures *above the foramen magnum*. The mnemonic device used to study the cord provides an excellent foundation for understanding the anatomy here (see A Summary of the Functional Anatomy of the Brain Stem, p. 95). To provide continuity, the same colors as in the cord have been applied here. Because vascular diseases so commonly involve the intracranial structures (unlike the cord), the major arterial supply is included.

Only tracts and nuclei with wide clinical application are shown in the illustrations. A brief review of the location and the function of the tracts and the nuclei of the cord and the brain stem precedes the respective sections.

Each plate shows a longitudinal and one or more cross sections of the nervous system, emphasizing the two steps in *the location of the lesion* outlined in Part I. The reader will note that some diseases are demonstrated better on the longitudinal view. If a neurogenic bladder occurs with the disease, the bladder is encircled.

At best, the profiles are schematic localizations of the lesions occurring in neurologic diseases on semidiagrammatic illustrations of the nervous system. Consequently, they are not expected fully to display the gross pathology of each disease. For example, the distortion and the hydrocephalus produced by tumors cannot be demonstrated.

The profiles, like pathologic specimens, are limited in that they can represent only one stage of a dynamic life process consisting of many stages. A few diseases are illustrated in two or more stages to dramatize this point.

Moreover, the plates represent only the more typical location of the disease process. It must be kept in mind that both the intensity and the location of the process will differ from case to case. Almost invariably, each neurologic case encountered in practice has some unique aspect. The more common variations are shown in selected disorders. To illustrate them all would require several volumes.

SECTION A

LESIONS BELOW THE FORAMEN MAGNUM

A Summary of the Functional Anatomy of the Spinal Cord

The basic anatomy of the spinal cord is visualized best as a stack of *reflex arcs* enclosed by *ascending sensory* and *descending motor tracts* (the white matter) connecting these arcs with cortical, cerebellar and brain-stem centers. The components and the functions of the reflex arc (sense organ, muscle, peripheral nerve, sensory root and horn, motor root and horn) are familiar to most students of neurology. The function of the tracts is understood more easily if they, too, are thought of as parts of "arcs," the intermediate portions of which rest in cortical, brain-stem and cerebellar centers.

The sensory root "feeds" information directly or indirectly to four sensory tracts with clinical significance:

1. Directly to the *posterior column*, transmitting proprioceptive sensation to the brain stem, where in turn it is relayed to the thalamus by secondary fibers and, finally, to the cortex by tertiary fibers.

2. Indirectly to the *lateral spinothalamic tract*, through secondary fibers, transmitting pain and temperature sensation to the thalamus.

3. Indirectly to the *ventral spinothalamic tract*, through secondary fibers, transmitting light-touch sensation to the thalamus.

4. Indirectly to the *spinocerebellar tracts,* through secondary fibers, providing the cerebellum with proprioceptive sense.

The fibers joining the spinothalamic tracts first must cross the cord via the *ventral commissure* near their site of origin.

The motor-horn cells are controlled by several descending tracts, but only the divisions of the pyramidal tract, *the lateral* and the *ventral columns,* have broad clinical application. They give us voluntary control.

The mnemonic device (p. 49) demonstrates adequately the relative positions of the various tracts in the cord.

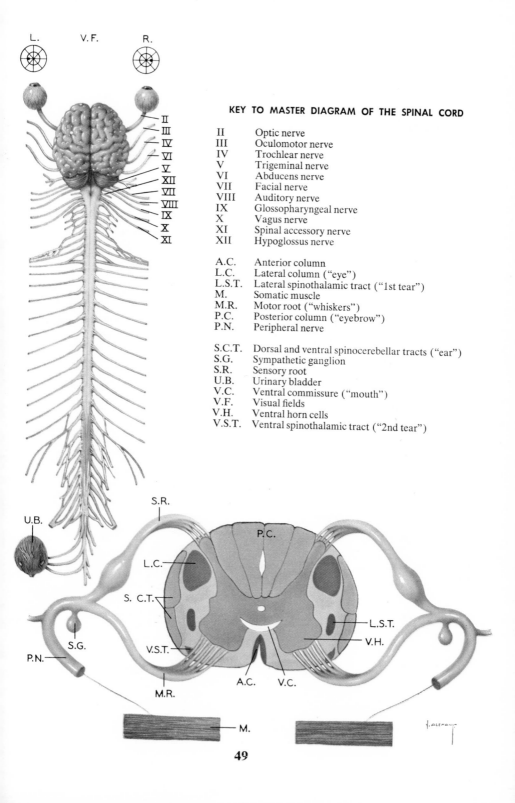

L.　V.F.　R.

KEY TO MASTER DIAGRAM OF THE SPINAL CORD

II	Optic nerve
III	Oculomotor nerve
IV	Trochlear nerve
V	Trigeminal nerve
VI	Abducens nerve
VII	Facial nerve
VIII	Auditory nerve
IX	Glossopharyngeal nerve
X	Vagus nerve
XI	Spinal accessory nerve
XII	Hypoglossus nerve
A.C.	Anterior column
L.C.	Lateral column ("eye")
L.S.T.	Lateral spinothalamic tract ("1st tear")
M.	Somatic muscle
M.R.	Motor root ("whiskers")
P.C.	Posterior column ("eyebrow")
P.N.	Peripheral nerve
S.C.T.	Dorsal and ventral spinocerebellar tracts ("ear")
S.G.	Sympathetic ganglion
S.R.	Sensory root
U.B.	Urinary bladder
V.C.	Ventral commissure ("mouth")
V.F.	Visual fields
V.H.	Ventral horn cells
V.S.T.	Ventral spinothalamic tract ("2nd tear")

S.R.

U.B.

P.C.

L.C.

S. C.T.

L.S.T.

S.G.

V.H.

P.N.

V.S.T.

A.C.　V.C.

M.R.

M.

Amyotrophic Lateral Sclerosis

A 34-year-old white male complained that he had had difficulty buttoning his clothes and had dropped things frequently during the past 3 months.

Neurologic examination disclosed weakness of flexion, extension, abduction and adduction of the fingers of both hands but more marked on the right; atrophy and fasciculations of the hypothenar and the interossei muscles bilaterally, and hyperactive biceps, patellar and Achilles reflexes.

Treatable Diseases To Be Ruled Out
Spinal cord tumor
Ruptured nucleus pulposus
Cervical spondylosis
Tuberculosis of the spinal column
Nutritional neuropathy
Syphilitic meningomyelitis

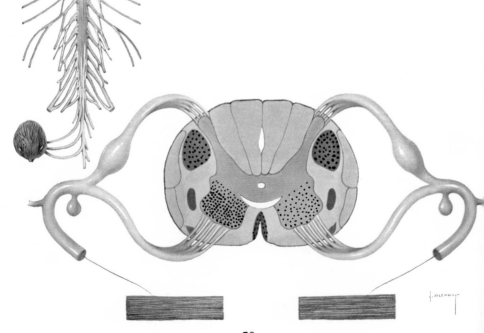

Amyotrophic Lateral Sclerosis

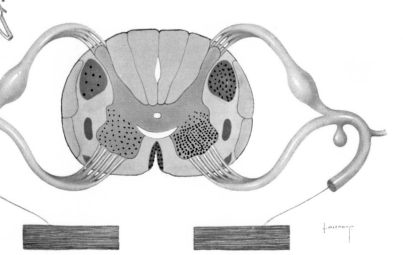

A 56-year-old Negro male complained of gradual on-set of weakness in the left extremities for the past 4 years. This had become more severe in the preceding 4 months, and, in addition, he had noted generalized twitching of the arms and the legs, marked weight loss and difficulty in climbing stairs.

Neurologic examination revealed marked emaciation with weakness, atrophy and fasciculations on all 4 extremities, but more marked on the left. The deep tendon reflexes were reduced throughout, but more so on the right. There was a left Babinski sign.

Treatable Diseases To Be Ruled Out

Spinal cord tumor
Ruptured nucleus pulposus
Cervical spondylosis
Tuberculosis of the spinal column
Nutritional neuropathy
Syphilitic meningomyelitis

Friedreich's Ataxia

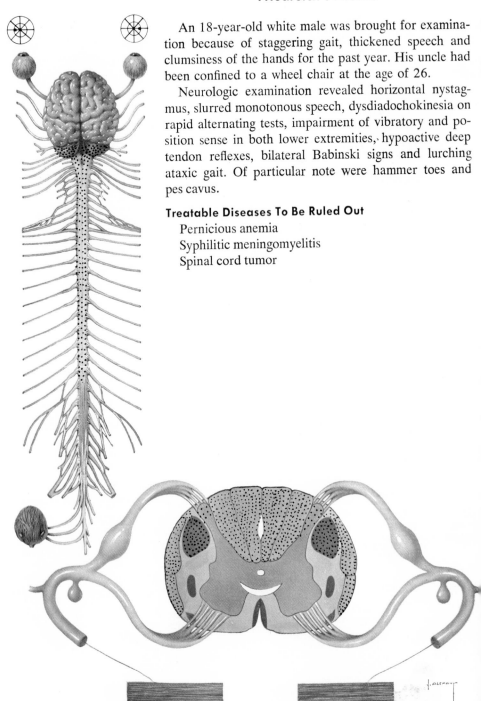

An 18-year-old white male was brought for examination because of staggering gait, thickened speech and clumsiness of the hands for the past year. His uncle had been confined to a wheel chair at the age of 26.

Neurologic examination revealed horizontal nystagmus, slurred monotonous speech, dysdiadochokinesia on rapid alternating tests, impairment of vibratory and position sense in both lower extremities, hypoactive deep tendon reflexes, bilateral Babinski signs and lurching ataxic gait. Of particular note were hammer toes and pes cavus.

Treatable Diseases To Be Ruled Out
Pernicious anemia
Syphilitic meningomyelitis
Spinal cord tumor

Multiple Sclerosis

A 32-year-old white female complained of intermittent weakness in the left arm and leg of 1-year's duration. This had cleared up almost completely 2 months prior to admission to the hospital, but only 1 week before this the left leg became so weak that she tripped on it frequently while walking. For the past 3 months she had experienced occasional incontinence of urine. At the age of 18 she had had an episode of diplopia that cleared up spontaneously.

Neurologic examination revealed temporal pallor of the left disk, weakness of the left hand grip, hyperactive reflexes of the left extremities, loss of superficial abdominal reflexes bilaterally and a left Babinski sign. She had a hemiplegic gait.

Treatable Diseases To Be Ruled Out
Pernicious anemia
Spinal cord tumor
Syphilitic meningomyelitis
Cervical spondylosis
Tuberculosis of the spinal column
NOTE: The speckled plaques are more recent.

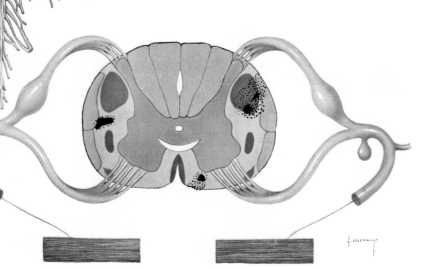

Multiple Sclerosis

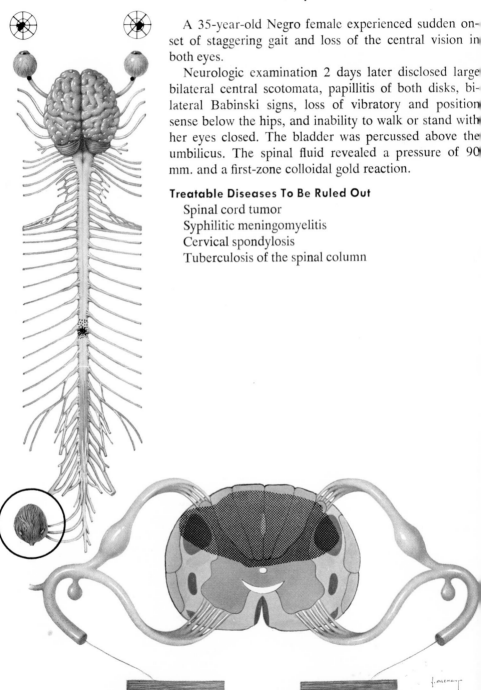

A 35-year-old Negro female experienced sudden onset of staggering gait and loss of the central vision in both eyes.

Neurologic examination 2 days later disclosed large bilateral central scotomata, papillitis of both disks, bilateral Babinski signs, loss of vibratory and position sense below the hips, and inability to walk or stand with her eyes closed. The bladder was percussed above the umbilicus. The spinal fluid revealed a pressure of 90 mm. and a first-zone colloidal gold reaction.

Treatable Diseases To Be Ruled Out
Spinal cord tumor
Syphilitic meningomyelitis
Cervical spondylosis
Tuberculosis of the spinal column

Multiple Sclerosis

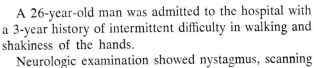

A 26-year-old man was admitted to the hospital with a 3-year history of intermittent difficulty in walking and shakiness of the hands.

Neurologic examination showed nystagmus, scanning speech, bilateral dysdiadochokinesia on rapid alternating tests, intention tremor of the arms and the legs, hyperactive deep tendon reflexes and bilateral Babinski signs.

He died 3 years later of a renal infection.

Treatable Diseases To Be Ruled Out
Spinal cord tumor
Syphilitic meningomyelitis
Cervical spondylosis
Tuberculosis of the spinal column
NOTE: The speckled plaques are more recent.

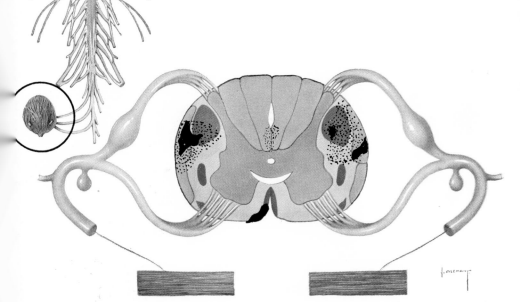

Pernicious Anemia

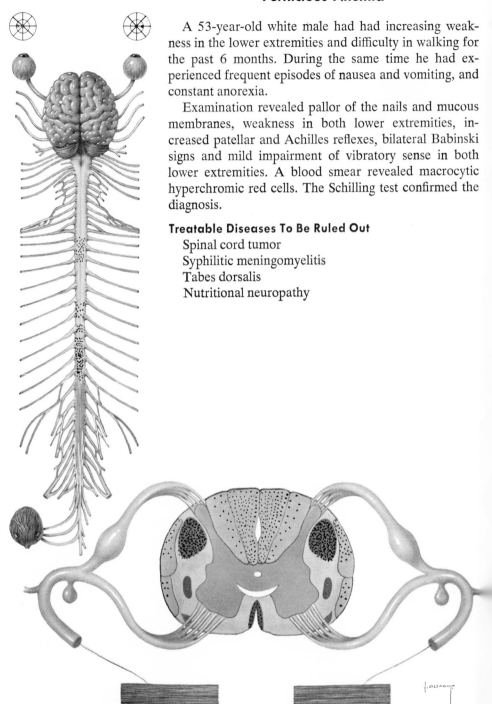

A 53-year-old white male had had increasing weakness in the lower extremities and difficulty in walking for the past 6 months. During the same time he had experienced frequent episodes of nausea and vomiting, and constant anorexia.

Examination revealed pallor of the nails and mucous membranes, weakness in both lower extremities, increased patellar and Achilles reflexes, bilateral Babinski signs and mild impairment of vibratory sense in both lower extremities. A blood smear revealed macrocytic hyperchromic red cells. The Schilling test confirmed the diagnosis.

Treatable Diseases To Be Ruled Out
Spinal cord tumor
Syphilitic meningomyelitis
Tabes dorsalis
Nutritional neuropathy

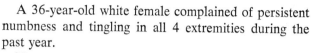

Pernicious Anemia

A 36-year-old white female complained of persistent numbness and tingling in all 4 extremities during the past year.

Neurologic examination disclosed loss of position and vibratory sense in both lower extremities, diminished patellar and Achilles reflexes, bilateral Babinski signs and a wide-based ataxia accentuated greatly by closing her eyes. A gastric analysis revealed histamine-resistant achlorhydria.

Treatable Diseases To Be Ruled Out
Spinal cord tumor
Syphilitic meningomyelitis
Tabes dorsalis
Nutritional neuropathy

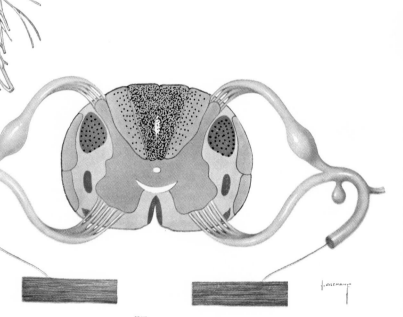

Progressive Muscular Atrophy

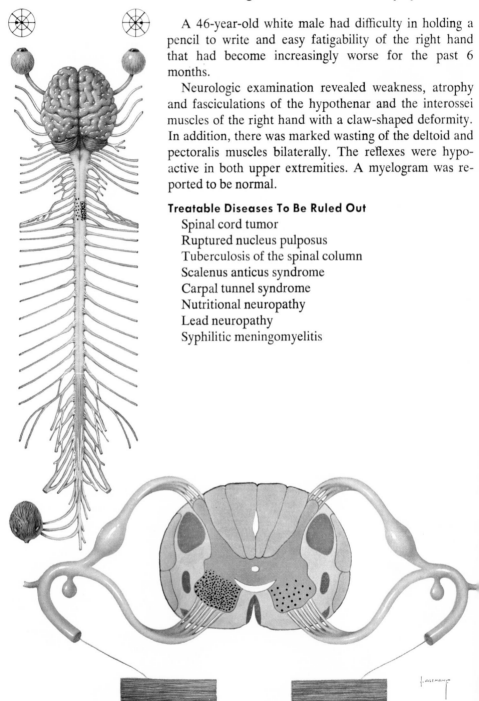

A 46-year-old white male had difficulty in holding a pencil to write and easy fatigability of the right hand that had become increasingly worse for the past 6 months.

Neurologic examination revealed weakness, atrophy and fasciculations of the hypothenar and the interossei muscles of the right hand with a claw-shaped deformity. In addition, there was marked wasting of the deltoid and pectoralis muscles bilaterally. The reflexes were hypoactive in both upper extremities. A myelogram was reported to be normal.

Treatable Diseases To Be Ruled Out

Spinal cord tumor
Ruptured nucleus pulposus
Tuberculosis of the spinal column
Scalenus anticus syndrome
Carpal tunnel syndrome
Nutritional neuropathy
Lead neuropathy
Syphilitic meningomyelitis

Syringomyelia

A 23-year-old nurse came to the emergency room for treatment of burns of her right hand and fingers sustained while using an autoclave. She denied any pain in her hand either during or after sustaining the burns.

Neurologic examination revealed bilateral loss of pain and temperature in the distribution of dermatomes C-4 to T-1 and a left Horner's syndrome. She had undergone surgery for a cleft palate at 2 years of age.

Treatable Diseases To Be Ruled Out
Spinal cord tumor
Cervical spondylosis
Bilateral cervical ribs
Nutritional neuropathy

NOTE: The shaded area represents the cavitation also.

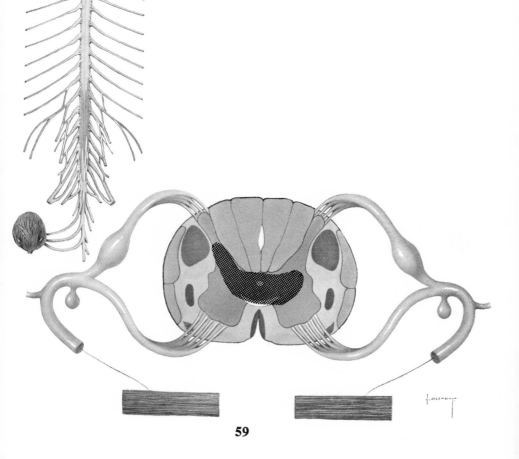

59

Syringomyelia

A 53-year-old bookkeeper with long-standing syringomyelia complained of progressive weakness in his right hand that was interfering with his work. He returned for examination because he feared losing his job.

Examination revealed weakness, atrophy and fasciculations of the interossei, the thenar and the hypothenar muscles of both hands, atrophy of both shoulder girdles, loss of pain and temperature and, to slight extent, vibratory sense between dermatomes C-2 and T-6 bilaterally. In addition, the deep tendon reflexes were increased in both lower extremities, and there was impairment of vibratory and position sense below the knee.

Treatable Diseases To Be Ruled Out
Spinal cord tumor
Cervical spondylosis
Bilateral cervical ribs
Nutritional neuropathy

NOTE: The shaded area represents the cavitation also.

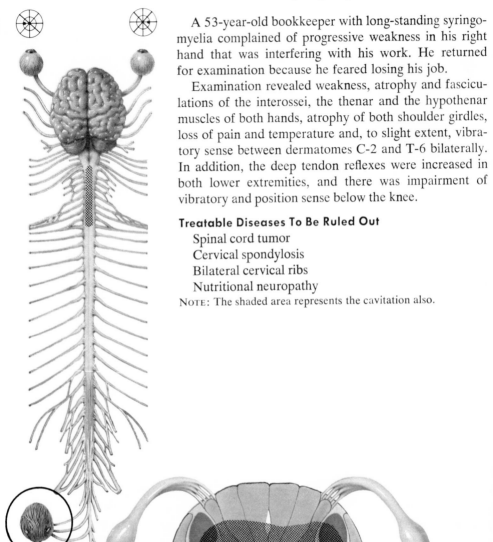

Werdnig-Hoffmann Disease

A young mother complained that her 8-month-old daughter was no longer able to crawl or sit up and had lost 3 pounds in the past month.

Neurologic examination disclosed generalized flaccidity and weakness, loss of deep tendon reflexes, and atrophy and fasciculations of all 4 extremities. Electromyography helped to establish the diagnosis.

Treatable Diseases To Be Ruled Out
Infectious polyneuritis
Lead neuropathy

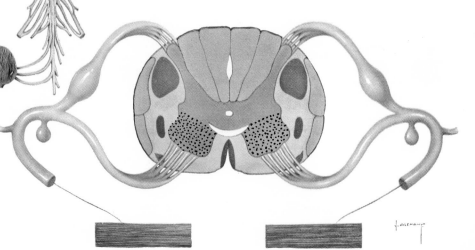

Epidural Abscess

A 48-year-old diabetic female developed rather suddenly severe backache and a girdlelike pain around the middle of her chest that was increased by sneezing. A chest roentgenogram and EKG at the time were within normal limits. On the second hospital day she complained of fever, chills and weakness in both legs.

Neurologic examination revealed weakness, hyperactive reflexes and Babinski signs in both lower extremities, diminished vibratory and position sense below the knees, and a sensory level at T-8 bilaterally. The urine contained many gram-positive cocci. On spinal puncture the Queckenstedt test revealed a complete block.

Treatable Diseases To Be Ruled Out
Tuberculoma
Spinal cord tumor

NOTE: The solid area represents the abscess; the speckled area, the effects of compression.

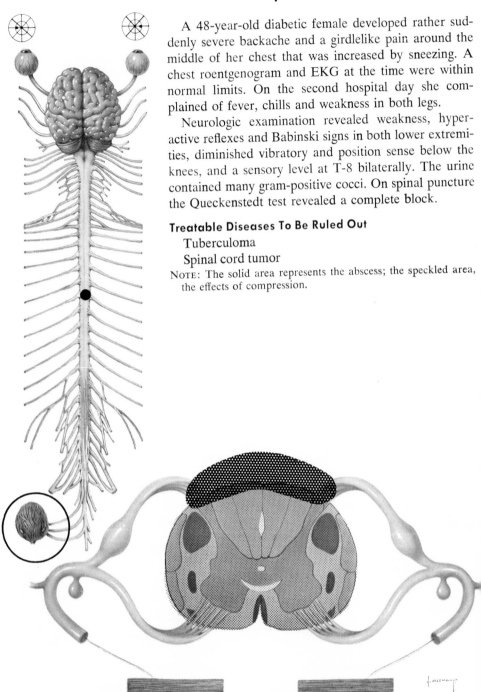

Herpes Zoster

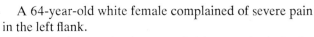

A 64-year-old white female complained of severe pain in the left flank.

Neurologic examination revealed hyperesthesia in the distribution of the left 12th thoracic nerve. Four days later she developed a bullous eruption in the left flank.

Treatable Diseases To Be Ruled Out
Renal calculi
Pyelonephritis
Extramedullary spinal cord tumor
Tuberculosis of the spinal column
Tabes dorsalis

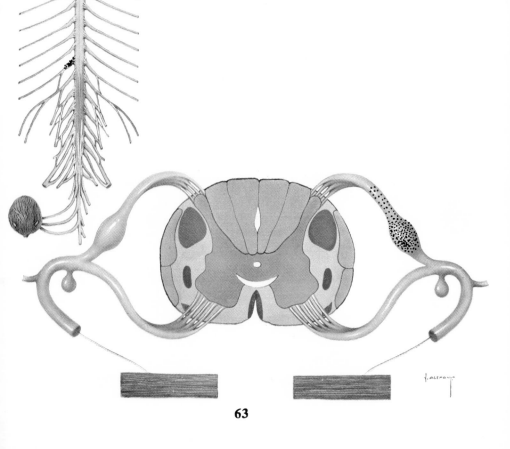

Infectious Polyneuritis

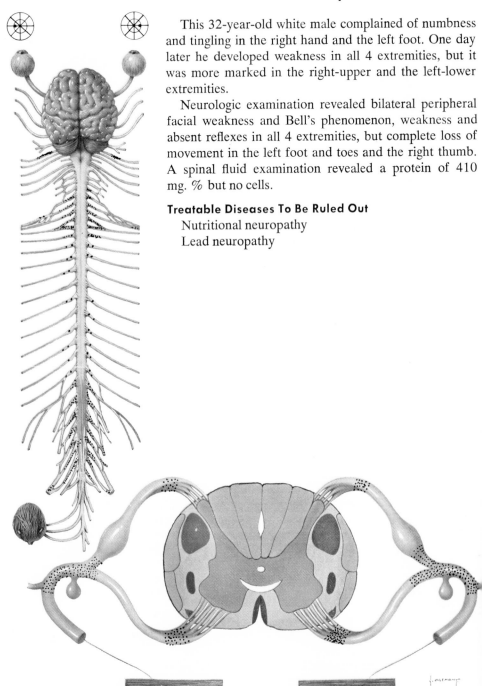

This 32-year-old white male complained of numbness and tingling in the right hand and the left foot. One day later he developed weakness in all 4 extremities, but it was more marked in the right-upper and the left-lower extremities.

Neurologic examination revealed bilateral peripheral facial weakness and Bell's phenomenon, weakness and absent reflexes in all 4 extremities, but complete loss of movement in the left foot and toes and the right thumb. A spinal fluid examination revealed a protein of 410 mg. % but no cells.

Treatable Diseases To Be Ruled Out
Nutritional neuropathy
Lead neuropathy

Infectious Polyneuritis

An 8-year-old white girl was admitted to the hospital because of increasing generalized weakness for 3 days. Two weeks prior to admission she had had a severe sore throat and fever lasting 2 days.

Neurologic examination disclosed slight nuchal rigidity, diffuse generalized weakness of the arms and the legs, shallow diaphragmatic breathing, absent deep tendon reflexes and bilateral foot drop. She was unable to rise to a sitting position without turning over on all fours. A spinal fluid protein was 230 mg. %. There were no cells.

Treatable Diseases To Be Ruled Out
Nutritional neuropathy
Lead neuropathy

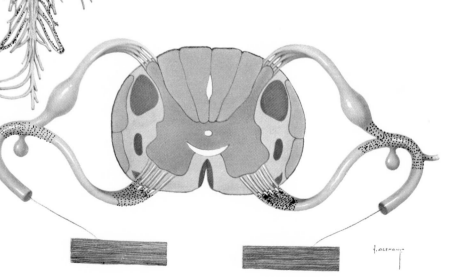

Poliomyelitis

A 9-year-old white girl had a sudden onset of diarrhea, vomiting and elevated temperature that was diagnosed as "viral gastroenteritis" and was treated by her local physician. Four days later she became very drowsy and was found to have a flaccid paralysis of her right arm and leg. She was admitted to the hospital with a diagnosis of "cerebrovascular accident."

A spinal fluid examination revealed 310 white cells per cu. mm. and a pressure of 280 mm. The consulting neurologist found hypoactive reflexes on all 4 extremities, in addition to the profound weakness of the right extremities. An electromyogram helped to establish the diagnosis.

Treatable Diseases To Be Ruled Out
Nutritional neuropathy
Infectious polyneuritis
Lead neuropathy
Bacterial meningitis
Epidural abscess

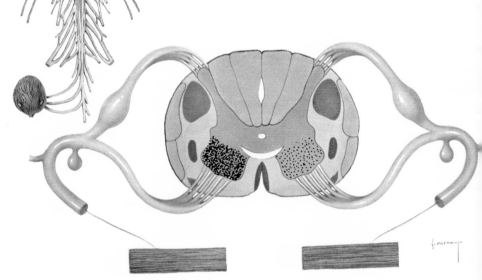

Poliomyelitis

A 7-year-old white boy developed fever, malaise, headache and nausea 3 days prior to admission to the hospital. On the day of admission the temperature rose again, and he developed pain in the neck and the lower extremities, and became very irritable.

Examination revealed nuchal rigidity, Kernig's sign, loss of the deep tendon reflexes in the lower extremities, but normal muscle power and gait. The spinal fluid contained 162 cells per cu. mm., most of them neutrophils. Within the next few days he developed extreme flaccid paralysis of the left leg, mild paralysis of the right leg and retention of urine.

Treatable Diseases To Be Ruled Out
Nutritional neuropathy
Infectious polyneuritis
Lead neuropathy
Bacterial meningitis
Epidural abscess

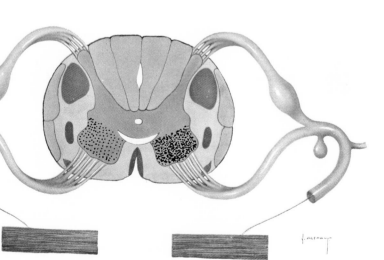

67

Syphilitic Meningomyelitis

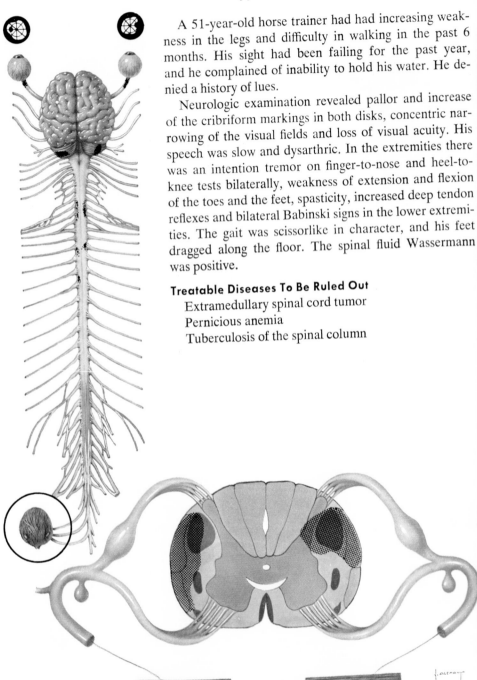

A 51-year-old horse trainer had had increasing weakness in the legs and difficulty in walking in the past 6 months. His sight had been failing for the past year, and he complained of inability to hold his water. He denied a history of lues.

Neurologic examination revealed pallor and increase of the cribriform markings in both disks, concentric narrowing of the visual fields and loss of visual acuity. His speech was slow and dysarthric. In the extremities there was an intention tremor on finger-to-nose and heel-to-knee tests bilaterally, weakness of extension and flexion of the toes and the feet, spasticity, increased deep tendon reflexes and bilateral Babinski signs in the lower extremities. The gait was scissorlike in character, and his feet dragged along the floor. The spinal fluid Wassermann was positive.

Treatable Diseases To Be Ruled Out

Extramedullary spinal cord tumor
Pernicious anemia
Tuberculosis of the spinal column

Syphilitic Meningomyelitis

A 38-year-old Negro male complained of increasing weakness in the right arm and leg and numbness and tingling of all 4 extremities for the past year. His wife noted that he had become depressed and disinterested in his business for the past 2 years. He had been treated for a generalized rash with large doses of penicillin 5 years prior to admission to the hospital.

Neurologic examination revealed Argyll Robertson pupils, weakness of the right-hand grip, atrophy and fasciculations of the deltoid and the interossei muscles on the right, increased right patellar and Achilles reflexes, a right Babinski sign, and mild loss of position and vibratory sense in the right arm and leg. There was loss of pinprick to T-1 on the left. He had difficulty in counting backward from 100 by 7's or 3's and had a poor attention span. The spinal fluid Wassermann was negative, but a Reiter protein was positive.

Treatable Diseases To Be Ruled Out
Extramedullary spinal cord tumor
Pernicious anemia
Tuberculosis of the spinal column

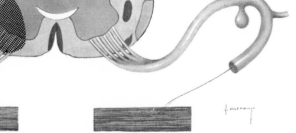

Tabes Dorsalis

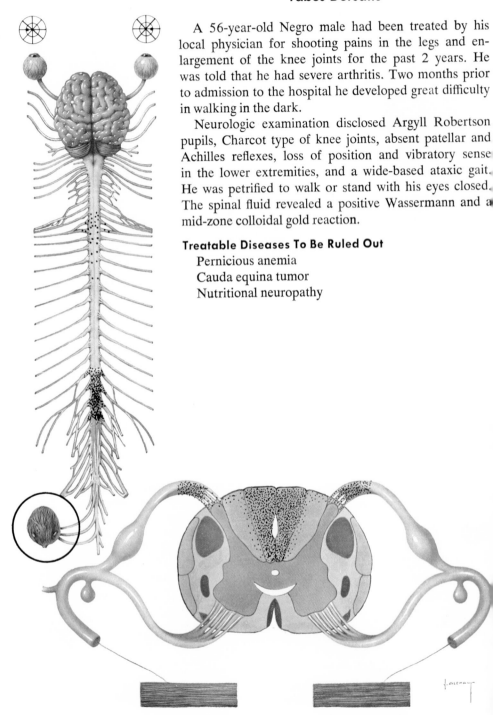

A 56-year-old Negro male had been treated by his local physician for shooting pains in the legs and enlargement of the knee joints for the past 2 years. He was told that he had severe arthritis. Two months prior to admission to the hospital he developed great difficulty in walking in the dark.

Neurologic examination disclosed Argyll Robertson pupils, Charcot type of knee joints, absent patellar and Achilles reflexes, loss of position and vibratory sense in the lower extremities, and a wide-based ataxic gait. He was petrified to walk or stand with his eyes closed. The spinal fluid revealed a positive Wassermann and a mid-zone colloidal gold reaction.

Treatable Diseases To Be Ruled Out
Pernicious anemia
Cauda equina tumor
Nutritional neuropathy

Extramedullary Spinal Cord Tumor
(Brown-Séquard Syndrome)

A 35-year-old Negro female had complained of pain in the left breast and weakness of the left leg for the past year. She had been told at another clinic 6 months prior to admission to the hospital that she had multiple sclerosis. One month prior to admission she was treated for an acute pyelonephritis by her local physician. Since then she had had occasional incontinence of urine.

Neurologic examination revealed weakness, spasticity, increased patellar and Achilles reflexes, and ankle clonus in the left leg. There were loss of vibratory and position sense to the hip on the left and loss of pain and temperature to T-7 on the right. A roentgenogram of the thoracic spine revealed erosion of the pedicles at T-5 and T-6.

Treatable Diseases To Be Ruled Out
Syphilitic meningomyelitis
Tuberculosis of the spinal column

NOTE: The dark area represents the tumor; the light area, the effects of compression.

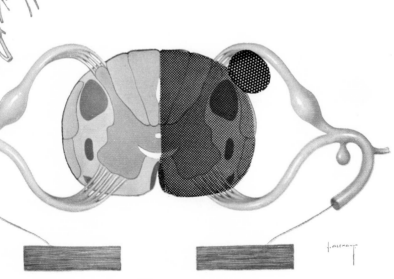

71

Extramedullary Spinal Cord Tumor
(High Cervical)

A 44-year-old Negro male had had pain in the right suboccipital and mastoid area for 8 months prior to admission to the hospital. Roentgenograms of the skull and the mastoids had been normal at that time. Three months prior to admission he developed persistent numbness and tingling in all 4 extremities.

Neurologic examination revealed hyperactive reflexes in all 4 extremities, bilateral Babinski signs, and impairment of vibratory and position sense below the clavicles, but more profound loss in the legs. A cervical myelogram confirmed the diagnosis.

Treatable Diseases To Be Ruled Out
Syphilitic meningomyelitis
Tuberculosis of the spinal column
Pernicious anemia
Platybasia
Ruptured nucleus pulposus
Cervical spondylosis

NOTE: The dark area represents the tumor; the light area, the effects of compression.

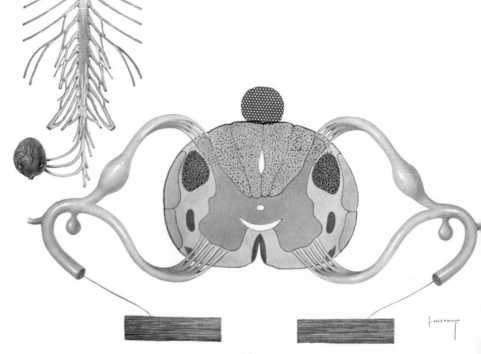

72

Extramedullary Spinal Cord Tumor

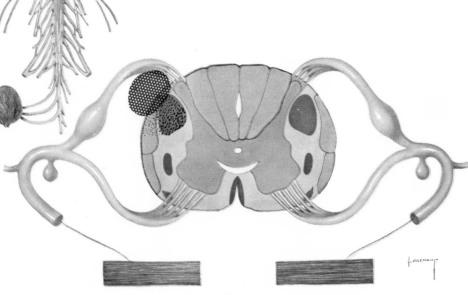

A 39-year-old obese housewife had complained of intermittent right-upper-quadrant pain for the past 6 months. Cholecystograms and pyelograms repeatedly had been normal. One week prior to admission to the hospital the pain became more constant and radicular in nature.

Neurologic examination revealed increased right patellar and Achilles reflexes, and a right Babinski sign. The spinal fluid protein was 114 mg. %. A myelogram confirmed the diagnosis.

Treatable Diseases To Be Ruled Out

Syphilitic meningomyelitis
Tuberculosis of the spinal column
Pernicious anemia
Ruptured nucleus pulposus

NOTE: The solid area represents the tumor; the speckled areas indicate the tracts or the nuclei involved by compression.

Extramedullary Spinal Cord Tumor

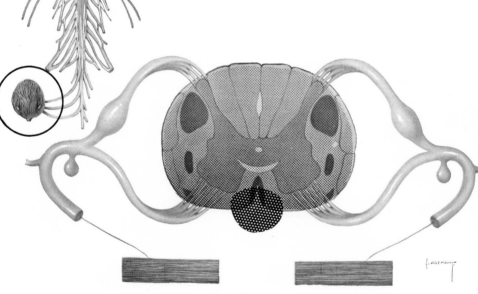

A 69-year-old white female had had a 2-year history of back pain that was diagnosed as osteoporosis, and she had been treated by her local physician. Eight months prior to admission to the hospital she developed progressive difficulty in walking and required the use of a cane. This, too, was attributed to osteoporosis. A Colles fracture of the left wrist brought her to the hospital.

Neurologic examination disclosed profound weakness, spasticity and hyperactive reflexes in both lower extremities, and bilateral Babinski signs. There was involuntary withdrawal of the legs to noxious stimuli. No pain or temperature was perceived below T-4 bilaterally, but there was exquisite pain sensation just above this. The myelogram revealed a complete block at T-3.

Treatable Diseases To Be Ruled Out
Syphilitic meningomyelitis
Tuberculosis of the spinal column
Pernicious anemia
Ruptured nucleus pulposus

NOTE: The dark area represents the tumor; the light areas indicate the tracts or the nuclei involved by compression.

74

Intramedullary Spinal Cord Tumor

A 44-year-old white female complained of progressive weakness in the lower extremities and difficulty in walking for the past 8 months. She had had urgency of urination for the past 3 months.

Neurologic examination disclosed weakness, spasticity, increased deep tendon reflexes and Babinski signs on both lower extremities. A sensory level was located at T-4 bilaterally, but there was no loss of pain or temperature below L-5 ("sacral sparing"). The spinal fluid protein was 140 mg. %. A myelogram revealed a filling defect at T-3, but the dye passed freely throughout the length of the spine.

Treatable Diseases To Be Ruled Out

See Extramedullary Spinal Cord Tumors.

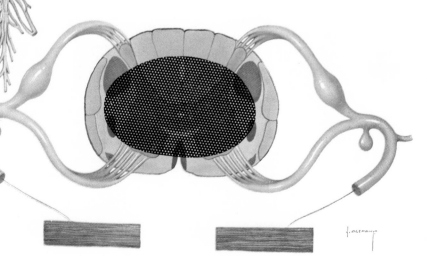

Cauda Equina Tumor

A 68-year-old Negro male was admitted to the urology service for chronic urinary retention. Cystoscopy failed to disclose bladder-neck obstruction. On careful questioning the patient related that, in the past year, he had had occasional severe pains in his low back that radiated down his left leg.

Neurologic examination revealed a positive straight-leg-raising test bilaterally, loss of the Achilles reflexes, and sacral anesthesia and analgesia. The spinal fluid protein was 90 mg. %. A myelogram confirmed the diagnosis.

Treatable Diseases To Be Ruled Out
Ruptured nucleus pulposus
Spondylolisthesis
Tuberculosis of the spine
Pelvic tumor

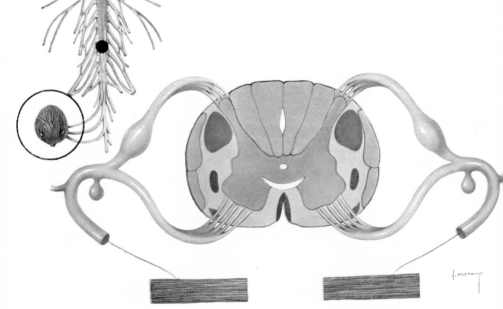

Metastatic Carcinoma

A 68-year-old white male with a 1-year history of back pain developed progressive weakness of the legs and difficulty in walking 3 months prior to admission to the hospital. Two weeks prior to admission he became incontinent of urine and feces.

Neurologic examination revealed weakness, spasticity, increased deep tendon reflexes and bilateral Babinski signs with a short-stepped spastic gait. There was a sensory level at L-1 on the left. On rectal examination the prostate was firm and nodular. A roentgenogram of the lower thoracic spine revealed increased density of T-11 and T-12 vertebrae.

Treatable Diseases To Be Ruled Out
Extramedullary spinal cord tumor
Tuberculosis of the spinal column
Syphilitic meningomyelitis

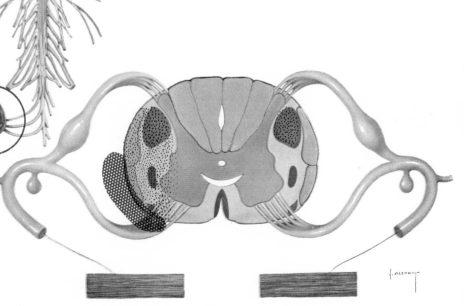

Anterior Spinal Artery Occlusion

A 48-year-old Negro female with a known history of lues had a sudden onset of weakness in the lower extremities.

Neurologic examination revealed flaccid paralysis of both lower extremities, bilateral Rossolimo signs and a sensory level at T-5 bilaterally.

Treatable Diseases To Be Ruled Out
Epidural abscess
Extramedullary spinal cord tumor
Tuberculoma
Syphilis

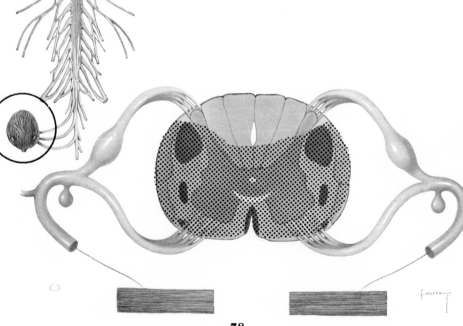

Compression Fracture of Spine

A 28-year-old Negro male was brought to the emergency ward unable to move all 4 extremities following an automobile accident.

Neurologic examination revealed flaccid paralysis of all 4 extremities and loss of deep tendon reflexes. The bladder was percussed above the umbilicus. A roentgenogram of the cervical spine revealed fractures of the 6th and the 7th cervical vertebrae. A spinal tap revealed a complete block. An operative decompression was performed. On examination 3 weeks later he had developed diffuse atrophy in the upper extremities and marked spasticity in the lower extremities.

Treatable Diseases To Be Ruled Out: None

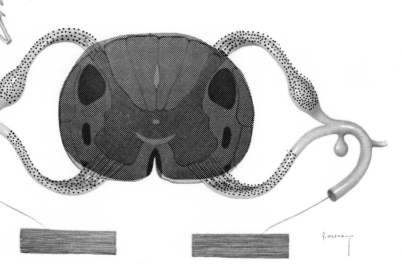

Cervical Spondylosis

A 47-year-old Polish laborer had had intermittent severe pain in both shoulders, especially at night, for the past year. For the past 3 months he had dragged his feet as he walked, and he was very unsteady at times, especially in the dark. Frequently his feet felt as if he were standing on hot pavement.

Neurologic examination disclosed mild atrophy and weakness of the left shoulder and the hand muscles, and hyperactive patellar and Achilles reflexes. There were loss of sensation in dermatomes C-5 and C-6 bilaterally and impairment of vibratory and position sense below the knees. A roentgenogram of the cervical spine revealed advanced osteoarthritic changes, and the cervical canal measured 12 mm. in diameter.

Treatable Diseases To Be Ruled Out
Tuberculosis of the spinal column
Ruptured nucleus pulposus
Extramedullary spinal cord tumor
Syphilitic meningomyelitis

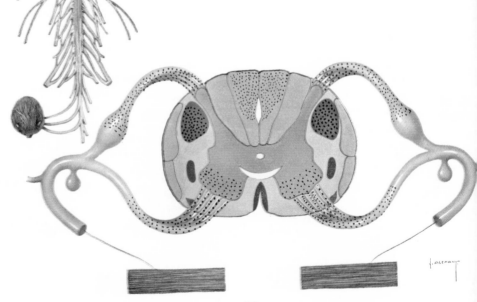

Osteoarthritis

A 49-year-old white male suddenly developed severe left precordial pain while swinging a golf club.

Neurologic examination revealed that the same pain could be reproduced by rotating to the right. An EKG was within normal limits. A roentgenogram of the thoracic spine demonstrated marked arthritic changes of the thoracic vertebrae.

Treatable Diseases To Be Ruled Out
Coronary insufficiency
Tuberculosis of the spinal column
Extramedullary spinal cord tumor
Tabes dorsalis

NOTE: The area of compression is speckled.

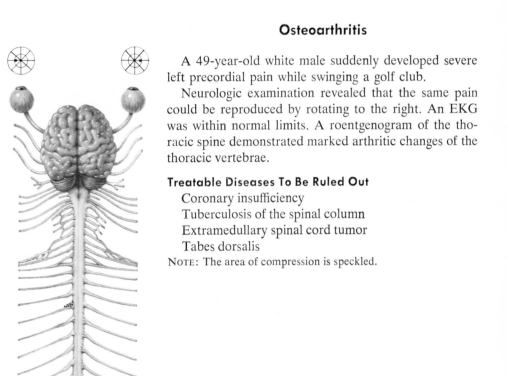

Ruptured Nucleus Pulposus
(Lumbar)

A 33-year-old Negro laborer developed severe lancinating pain that radiated down the posterior aspect of the left thigh while he was lifting a heavy steel beam.

Neurologic examination disclosed slight lumbar scoliosis to the right, weakness of dorsiflexion of the left toes, diminished left Achilles reflex, and hypalgesia of the lateral aspect of the left lower leg and foot, including the dorsolateral surface of the big toe. The pain was reproduced by rotating the spine to the right and bending forward, on straight-leg-raising to 60° (Lasègue's sign), on percussion of the 5th lumbar vertebra, and by bilateral jugular compression. A lumbar myelogram confirmed the diagnosis.

Treatable Diseases To Be Ruled Out
Cauda equina tumor
Tuberculosis of the spinal column
Pelvic tumors
Spondylolisthesis

NOTE: The transverse view of the cervical cord is used to demonstrate pathology that actually occurs in the lumbar cord.

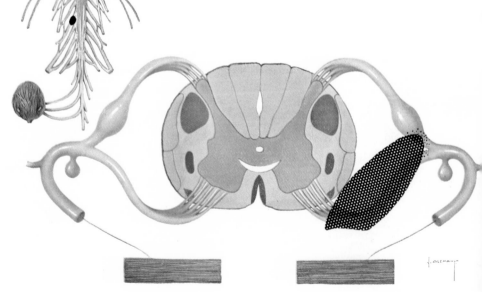

Ruptured Nucleus Pulposus
(Lateral Cervical)

A 63-year-old Negro male complained of severe lancinating pain that radiated down the medial aspect of the right arm and forearm. The pain was relieved by lying down but increased by coughing or sneezing. It did not seem to be brought on by exercise.

Neurologic examination revealed hypesthesia and hypalgesia of the right index and middle fingers, and fasciculations in the right triceps. Marked tenderness was elicited on percussion of the 7th and the 8th cervical vertebrae. A roentgenogram of the cervical spine revealed marked osteoarthritic changes and narrowing of the 3 lower cervical intervertebral spaces. There was remarkable relief of symptoms and signs after 3 weeks of cervical traction.

Treatable Diseases To Be Ruled Out
Spinal cord tumor
Tuberculosis of the spinal column
Scalenus anticus syndrome
Pancoast tumor
Carpal tunnel syndrome

NOTE: The solid area represents a protruded disk; the speckled area, the effects of compression.

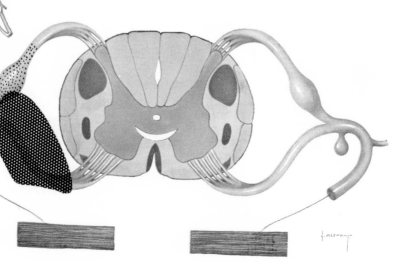

Ruptured Nucleus Pulposus
(Median Cervical)

A 54-year-old obese white male had a 2-week history of weakness, numbness and tingling in both upper extremities. One day prior to admission to the hospital he suddenly developed severe pain in the lateral aspect of the left shoulder.

Neurologic examination revealed weakness, atrophy and fasciculations of the shoulder girdle bilaterally, diminished left biceps reflex, loss of the superficial abdominal reflexes, hyperactive patellar and Achilles reflexes, and a left Babinski sign. A roentgenogram of the cervical spine revealed moderate osteoarthritic changes and narrowing of the interspace at C-5 to C-6. A cervical myelogram confirmed the diagnosis.

Treatable Diseases To Be Ruled Out

Spinal cord tumor
Tuberculosis of the spinal column
Cervical spondylosis
Syphilitic meningomyelitis

NOTE: The solid area represents a protruded disk; the speckled area, the effects of compression.

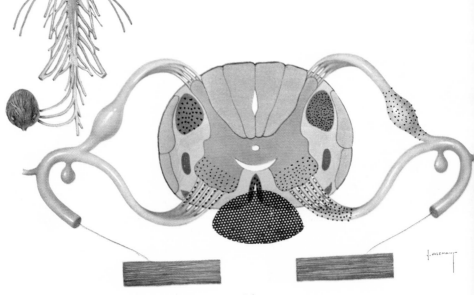

Tuberculosis of the Spinal Column

A 56-year-old white female with a 6-month history of neck pain complained of progressive weakness, paresthesia and loss of feeling in both hands of 2 months' duration. For the past month she had experienced difficulty in walking and especially in climbing stairs.

Neurologic examination revealed tenderness on percussion and palpation of the lower cervical spines; weakness, atrophy and fasciculations of the hypothenar and the interossei muscles bilaterally; weakness, increased deep tendon reflexes and Babinski signs in both lower extremities, and loss of sensation in dermatomes C-7, C-8 and T-1 bilaterally. A roentgenogram of the cervical spine revealed a moth-eaten appearance of the lower cervical vertebrae and collapse of the 7th cervical vertebra. A PPD No. 1 skin test was markedly positive. Bone biopsy was diagnostic.

Treatable Diseases To Be Ruled Out
Extramedullary spinal cord tumor
Cervical spondylosis
Syphilitic meningomyelitis
NOTE: The speckled areas represent the effects of compression.

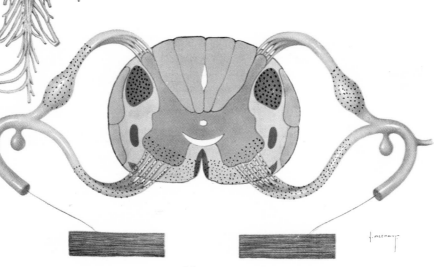

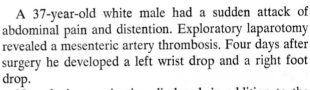

Periarteritis Nodosa

A 37-year-old white male had a sudden attack of abdominal pain and distention. Exploratory laparotomy revealed a mesenteric artery thrombosis. Four days after surgery he developed a left wrist drop and a right foot drop.

Neurologic examination disclosed, in addition to the above findings, hypesthesia and hypalgesia in the distribution of the left radial and the right common peroneal nerves. A muscle biopsy confirmed the diagnosis.

Treatable Diseases To Be Ruled Out

Nutritional neuropathy

Lead neuropathy

NOTE: The lesions are located in the peripheral portions of the nerves spotted on the longitudinal view.

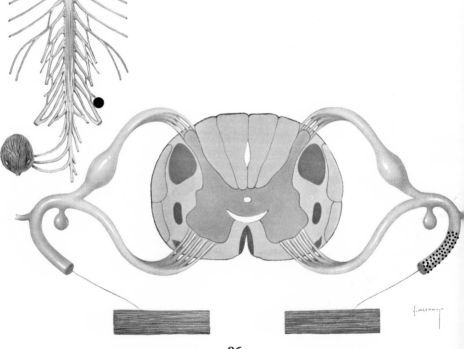

Diabetic Neuropathy

A 58-year-old white male complained of weakness, numbness and tingling in both hands for the past 4 weeks.

Neurologic examination revealed weakness of adduction and flexion of the fingers of both hands, atrophy of the small hand muscles bilaterally, loss of the Achilles reflexes and diminished vibratory sense in the lower extremities. A 2-hour postprandial blood sugar was 250 mg. %.

Treatable Diseases To Be Ruled Out
Nutritional neuropathy
Lead neuropathy

NOTE: The lesions are located in the peripheral portions of the nerves spotted on the longitudinal view.

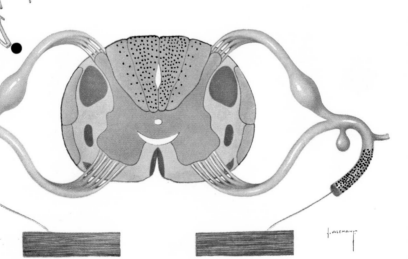

87

Lead Neuropathy

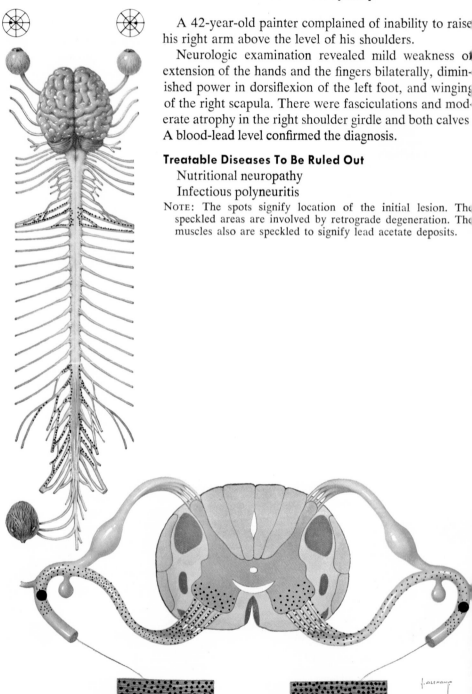

A 42-year-old painter complained of inability to raise his right arm above the level of his shoulders.

Neurologic examination revealed mild weakness of extension of the hands and the fingers bilaterally, diminished power in dorsiflexion of the left foot, and winging of the right scapula. There were fasciculations and moderate atrophy in the right shoulder girdle and both calves. A blood-lead level confirmed the diagnosis.

Treatable Diseases To Be Ruled Out

Nutritional neuropathy

Infectious polyneuritis

NOTE: The spots signify location of the initial lesion. The speckled areas are involved by retrograde degeneration. The muscles also are speckled to signify lead acetate deposits.

88

Nutritional Neuropathy

A 54-year-old white male underwent a subtotal gastrectomy for a peptic ulcer. His postoperative course was stormy, and oral intake was poor for the first month. Approximately 5 weeks after surgery he suddenly developed weakness in all 4 extremities and loss of feeling in both hands.

Neurologic examination revealed marked weakness, atrophy and diminished deep tendon reflexes of all 4 extremities. There were glove-and-stocking hypesthesia and hypalgesia, and almost total loss of vibratory sense below the knees. The gait was high stepping in character. After a week of thiamine and nicotinic acid therapy there was a remarkable improvement in both symptoms and signs.

Treatable Disease To Be Ruled Out

Infectious polyneuritis

NOTE: The lesions are located in the peripheral portions of the nerves spotted on the longitudinal view.

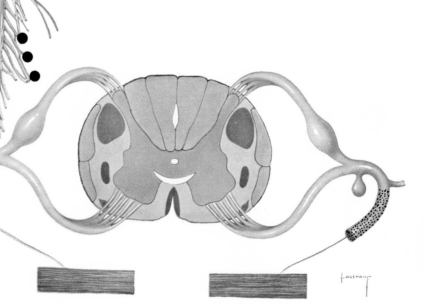

Peroneal Muscular Atrophy

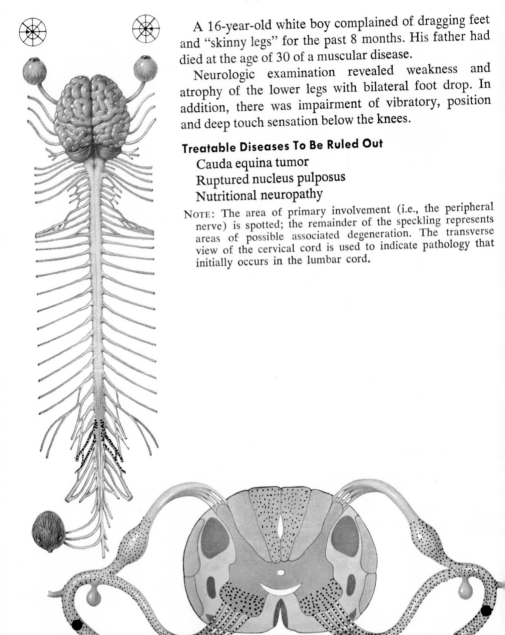

A 16-year-old white boy complained of dragging feet and "skinny legs" for the past 8 months. His father had died at the age of 30 of a muscular disease.

Neurologic examination revealed weakness and atrophy of the lower legs with bilateral foot drop. In addition, there was impairment of vibratory, position and deep touch sensation below the knees.

Treatable Diseases To Be Ruled Out

Cauda equina tumor

Ruptured nucleus pulposus

Nutritional neuropathy

NOTE: The area of primary involvement (i.e., the peripheral nerve) is spotted; the remainder of the speckling represents areas of possible associated degeneration. The transverse view of the cervical cord is used to indicate pathology that initially occurs in the lumbar cord.

Porphyria

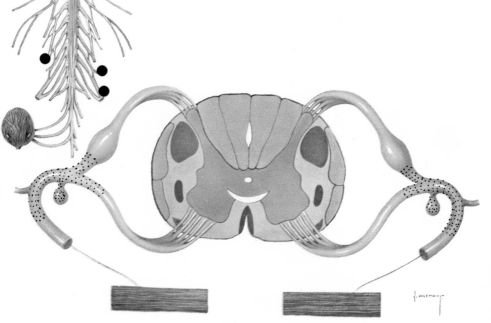

A 29-year-old white male had an episode of colicky right-lower-quadrant pain and nausea, and an emergency appendectomy was performed. The appendix was reported to be normal, and the pain continued, sometimes shifting to other parts of the abdomen. Two weeks after hospitalization a neurologist was consulted because the patient had become delirious and complained of severe pain in the arms and the legs.

Neurologic examination revealed marked weakness and atrophy of the muscles of all 4 extremities, and mild tenderness of the peripheral nerve trunks. It was difficult to examine adequately for an organic mental disorder, but there seemed to be impairment of judgment and lack of emotional control. The urine revealed large amounts of porphobilinogen.

Treatable Diseases To Be Ruled Out
Nutritional neuropathy
Infectious polyneuritis
Lead neuropathy

NOTE: The lesions are located in the peripheral portions of the nerves spotted on the longitudinal view.

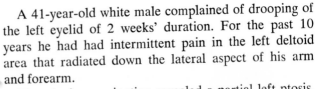

Scalenus Anticus Syndrome

A 41-year-old white male complained of drooping of the left eyelid of 2 weeks' duration. For the past 10 years he had had intermittent pain in the left deltoid area that radiated down the lateral aspect of his arm and forearm.

Neurologic examination revealed a partial left ptosis, a small left pupil and loss of the ciliospinal reflex on the left. There were slight weakness of the left-hand grip and a diminished left biceps reflex. The left radial pulse was obliterated on pulling the arm back and downward.

Treatable Diseases To Be Ruled Out

Spinal cord tumor
Ruptured nucleus pulposus
Pancoast tumor
Tuberculosis of spinal column
Cervical spondylosis

NOTE: The scalenus anticus muscle is sketched in.

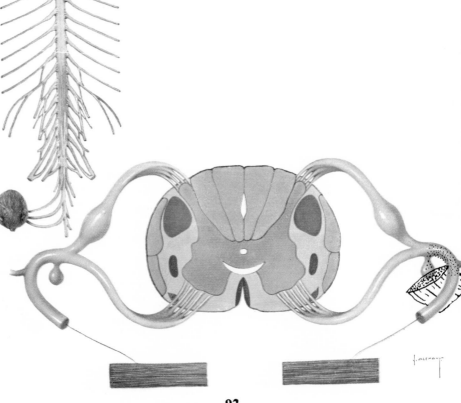

Progressive Muscular Dystrophy

A 14-year-old boy presented himself for examination because his friends teased him about the way his shoulders "stuck out in back." On questioning it was found that for the past year he had noted weakness in his arms and legs, so much so that he was forced to drop off the swimming team. His uncle had died at an early age of a muscular disease.

Neurologic examination disclosed tapir lips, pole neck, symmetric weakness and atrophy of the muscles of the shoulder girdle, the hips and the thighs. He had a waddling gait, and there was a definite pelvic tilt. A muscle biopsy was diagnostic.

Treatable Diseases To Be Ruled Out
Lead neuropathy
Myasthenia gravis

NOTE: The proximal muscles of the extremities involved most in the dystrophy are drawn in.

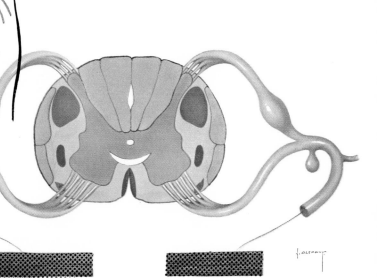

SECTION B

LESIONS ABOVE THE FORAMEN MAGNUM

A Summary of the Functional Anatomy of the Brain Stem

The maze of tracts and nuclei in the brain stem need not frighten students of anatomy. Those tracts and nuclei with concrete clinical application are almost as few as those in the cord. In fact, were it not for the addition of the special sensory nerves and nuclei, and the extrapyramidal system, for clinical purposes the brain stem might be regarded as a continuation of the cord. The strangeness of this mass begins to disappear when one recognizes that the brain stem possesses the same segmental structure as the cord. The "reflex arcs" and the major tracts of the cord have anatomic, or at least functional, corollaries in the brain stem.

1. The *crossed pyramidal tracts* (lateral columns) are crossed from their lateral position and lie at the base of the brain stem (all sections).

2. The posterior column terminates in the nuclei gracilis and cuneatus, but its function is continued in secondary fibers that cross to assume a midline, perpendicular position as the *medial lemniscus,* just above the pyramidal tract (Sec. 1). At higher levels, the medial lemniscus assumes a horizontal position (Secs. 2 & 3).

3. The *spinothalamic tracts* join each other and eventually join the medial lemniscus (Sec. 2) to terminate in the thalamus, but do not cross in the brain stem, as the contributing fibers to these tracts already have accomplished this near their point of origin in the cord.

4. The spinocerebellar tracts terminate in the cerebellum after passing through the medulla (Sec. 1). The dorsal spinocerebellar tract becomes a part of the *restiform body* (Sec. 1) before accomplishing this.

Farther up in the brain stem, an efferent cerebellar tract—the *brachium conjunctivum*—takes the relative position of the restiform body (Sec. 2) and then crosses to join the red nucleus (Sec. 3).

5. The sensory roots are joined into one big root of the *trigeminal nerve* (V) supplying the face and the forehead. Within the brain stem important parts of this root terminate in the *nucleus V* via the *spinal tract V* (Secs. 1 & 2). These are in the same relative position as their spinal cord counterparts (Lissauer tract, substantia gelatinosa). Secondary fibers from these structures cross and form the *trigemino-thalamic tracts* (Secs. 2 & 3) connecting with the thalamus.

6. The anterior horn cells and motor roots continue in the brain stem but are "shifted" upward and toward the mid-line by the underlying pyrami-

dal tracts, the medial lemniscus and other structures.* The "anterior horn cells" are represented as the *XII, XI, X, IX motor nuclei* in the medulla (Sec. 1); as the *VII, VI, V motor nuclei* in the pons (Sec. 2); and as the *IV* and *III motor nuclei* in the mid-brain (Sec. 3). Adjacent to some of these "somatic" motor nuclei are "visceral" *motor nuclei* (X, IX, VII, III) for autonomic functions. However, other than the *Edinger-Westphal nucleus* (III) serving the intrinsic muscles of the eyes, there is little clinical application for these "special" motor nuclei. Therefore, they have not been illustrated. Because they are at intermediate levels, motor nerves IV, IX, XI also are not illustrated in these Sections.

Thus far, the anatomy of the brain stem clearly is similar to the cord. The important additions are as follows:

1. *The Special Sensory Nerves and Nuclei*
   A. *The solitary nuclei* and *tracts* (taste) in the medulla, of so little practical application that they are not illustrated
   B. The *cochlear* and the *vestibular nerves* (VIII) and *nuclei* (Sec. 1), of greatest clinical importance in cerebellopontine angle tumors and aneurysms. An important vestibular pathway—the *medial longitudinal fasciculus* —because of its clinical application (e.g., multiple sclerosis), is included in the plates.
   C. The *optic nerves* (II), *chiasma* and *tracts* surrounding the hind portion of the diencephalon, of greatest practical significance in tumors and aneurysms in the sellar area (Sec. 4).
      The cortical connections (optic radiations, calcarine cortex) are important in temporal and occipital lobe space-taking lesions.
   D. The *olfactory bulbs* (I) and *tracts* in the forebrain, of importance in sphenoid ridge, olfactory groove and frontal lobe tumors.

2. *The Extrapyramidal System*
   Perhaps of less practical importance from a diagnostic standpoint, but anatomically more complex, are the extrapyramidal nuclei and tracts of the diencephalon and the mid-brain. Included in the plates are the *red nucleus* and the *substantia nigra* (Sec. 3); the *putamen*; the *globus pallidus* and the *caudate nucleus* (Sec. 4). These are involved most commonly in disease of this system.

To remind the reader how complex the anatomy of the brain stem can be presented, a list of brain-stem nuclei, tracts and regions with obscure or rare clinical application follows. These need concern only the neurologic specialist; therefore, they are not represented in the plates. It is important to note that a large portion of the brain stem is composed of fibers inter-

* Motor nuclei X (ambiguus) and VII do not assume this exact position, for, while they are elevated, they remain lateral.

connecting and co-ordinating the function of cortical, brain-stem and cerebellar centers.

1. Accessory olives
2. Arcuate nucleus
3. Hypothalamic nuclei
4. Inferior colliculus
5. Lateral lemniscus
6. Pontine fibers and nuclei
7. Reticulospinal tracts
8. Rhinencephalon
9. Subthalamic nucleus
10. Superior olive
11. Tectospinal tract
12. Tegmentum of mid-brain
13. Thalamic nuclei
14. Thalamo-rubro-olivary tract
15. Trapezoid body

Key to Master Diagram of the Brain

Each section of the brainstem is a composite of several sections, allowing for representation of those neuroanatomic structures with broadest clinical application.

I	Olfactory bulb	I.C.A.	Internal carotid artery
II	Optic nerve	I.O.	Inferior oblique muscle
III	Oculomotor nerve	I.O.	Inferior olive
IV	Trochlear nerve	I.R.	Inferior rectus muscle
V	Trigeminal nerve	L.P.S.	Levator palpebrae supe-
V_1	Ophthalmic division of		rioris muscle
	trigeminal nerve	M.B.	Mammillary bodies
V_2	Maxillary division of	M.C.A.	Middle cerebral artery
	trigeminal nerve	M.L.	Medial lemniscus
VI	Abducens nerve	M.L.F.	Medial longitudinal
VII	Facial nerve		fasciculus
c. VIII	Cochlear nerve	M.R.	Medial rectus muscle
v. VIII	Vestibular nerve	O.C.	Optic chiasma
IX	Glossopharyngeal nerve	O.L.	Occipital lobe
X	Vagus nerve	O.T.	Optic tract
XI	Spinal accessory nerve	P.	Putamen
XII	Hypoglossus nerve	P.C.	Posterior communicating
			artery
A.C.	Anterior communicating	P.C.A.	Posterior cerebral artery
	artery	P.G.	Pituitary gland
A.C.A.	Anterior cerebral artery	P.I.C.A.	Posterior inferior cere-
A.N.	Ambiguus nucleus		bellar artery
A.S.A.	Anterior spinal artery	P.T.	Pyramidal tract
B.A.	Basilar artery	R.B.	Restiform body
B.C.	Brachium conjunctivium	R.N.	Red nucleus
B.P.C.	Basis pedunculi cerebri	S.N.	Substantia nigra
C.C.	Corpus callosum	S.R.	Superior rectus muscle
C.H.	Cerebellar hemisphere	S.S.S.	Superior sagittal sinus
C.N.	Caudate nucleus	S.T.	Spinothalamic tract
D.	Dura	S.T.V.	Spinal tract of the
D.C.N.	Dorsal cochlear nucleus		trigeminal nerve
E.R.	External rectus muscle	T.L.	Temporal lobe
F.L.	Frontal lobe	T.T.	Trigemino-thalamic tract
F.M.	Muscles supplied by the	V.A.	Vertebral artery
	facial nerve	V.C.	Vermis cerebelli
G.F.	Genu of the facial nerve	V.C.N.	Ventral cochlear nucleus
G.P.	Globus pallidus	V.F.	Visual fields
I.C.	Internal capsule	V.N.	Vestibular nuclei

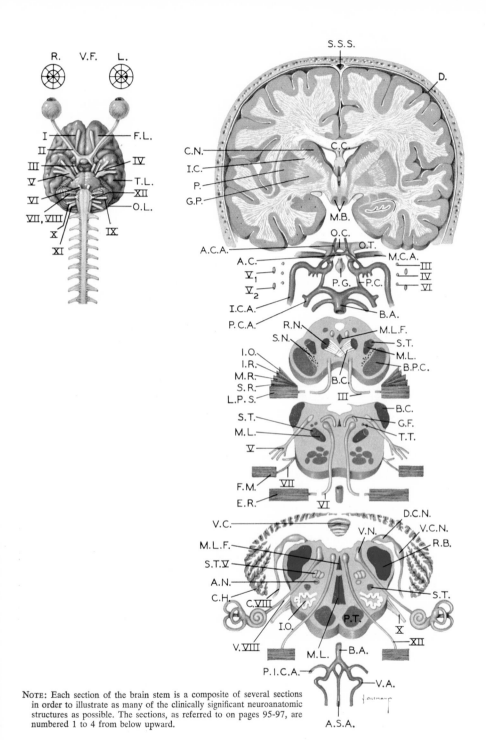

NOTE: Each section of the brain stem is a composite of several sections in order to illustrate as many of the clinically significant neuroanatomic structures as possible. The sections, as referred to on pages 95-97, are numbered 1 to 4 from below upward.

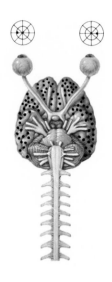

Alzheimer's Disease

A 65-year-old white female was admitted to the hospital after a 3-year history of an insidious onset of forgetfulness and impairment of judgment, with occasional acute episodes of disorientation in time and place. For 3 months prior to admission she had required frequent assistance with activities of daily living and was incontinent of urine.

Neurologic examination revealed marked disorientation in time and space, mixed aphasia, apraxia, pathologic mouth-opening responses, a grasp reflex on the right, and hyperactive reflexes of all 4 extremities, greater on the right. A pneumoencephalogram revealed marked dilatation of the entire ventricular system.

Treatable Diseases To Be Ruled Out
Space-taking lesions of the cerebrum
General paresis
Bromide intoxication

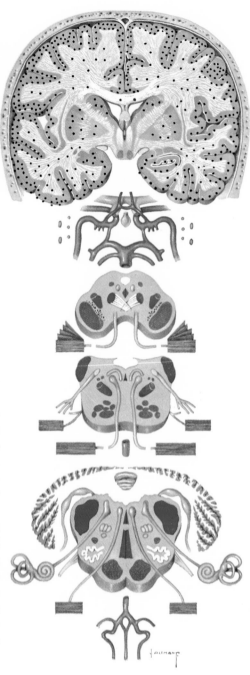

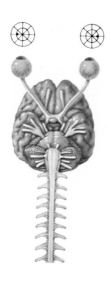

Bulbar Amyotrophic Lateral Sclerosis

A 38-year-old trumpet player had had difficulty in positioning his lips to play for the past 2 months. He also had noted difficulty in swallowing.

Neurologic examination revealed weakness, atrophy and fasciculations bilaterally in the face, tongue, sternocleidomastoid and the trapezius muscles, bulbar speech, and hyperactive reflexes of all 4 extremities.

Treatable Diseases To Be Ruled Out
Chordoma
Myasthenia gravis
Vertebral-basilar insufficiency
Syphilitic meningitis
Platybasia

NOTE: The facial nuclei are drawn in schematically to indicate that they, too, are involved.

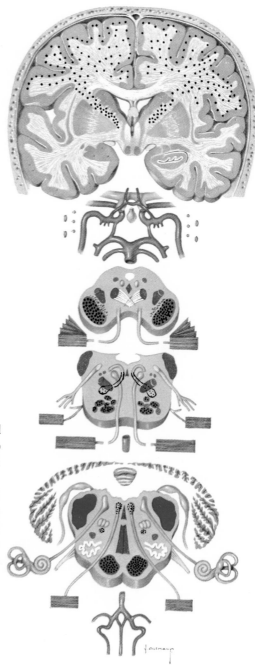

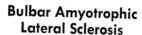

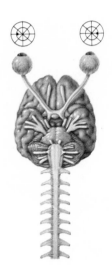

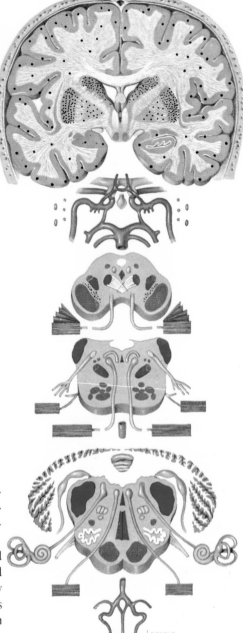

Huntington's Chorea

A 39-year-old white male complained of involuntary lurching movements of his arms and difficulty in walking.

Neurologic examination disclosed choreiform movements of the arms and the face; grotesque, clownish gait; slow mentation and poor attention span. His father had died in a mental institution at the age of 45.

Treatable Diseases To Be Ruled Out

Phenothiazine intoxication
Wilson's disease
Paralysis agitans

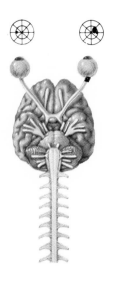

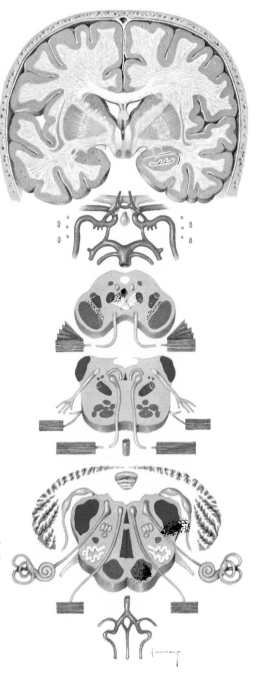

Multiple Sclerosis (Bulbar)

A 29-year-old white male had had intermittent staggering gait, dizziness and double vision for the past year. One week prior to admission to the hospital he developed a blind spot in his left visual field.

Neurologic examination revealed a left paracentral scotoma, disconjugate lateral gaze, nystagmus on left lateral gaze, perceptive deafness on the left, dysdiadochokinesia and an intention tremor of the left upper extremity, a wide-based ataxic gait and hyperactive reflexes in the right extremities.

Treatable Diseases To Be Ruled Out
Syphilitic meningitis
Tuberculous meningitis
Cerebellar abscess
Cerebellopontine angle tumor
Vertebral aneurysm
Vertebral-basilar insufficiency
Platybasia

NOTE: The speckled plaques are more recent.

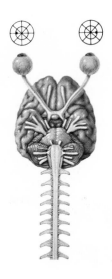

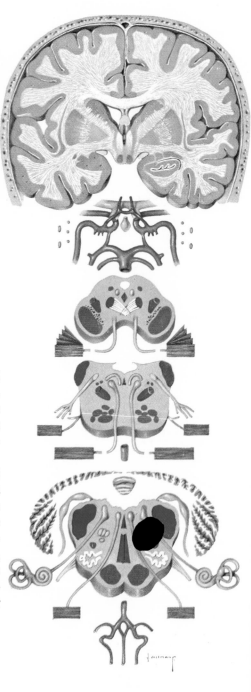

Syringobulbia

A 38-year-old white female had had
paroxysmal left facial pain for 2 years.
Injection technic failed to relieve the
pain. Two months prior to admission
to the hospital she developed hoarse-
ness and noisy breathing.

Neurologic examination disclosed
absent left corneal reflex, hypalgesia
of the left face and forehead, nystagmus
on left lateral gaze, deviation of the
uvula to the right, atrophy and fasciculations of the left side of the tongue,
loss of pain and temperature over the
right shoulder girdle and the right upper extremity, and an intention tremor
of the left upper extremity.

Treatable Diseases To Be Ruled Out
Cerebellopontine angle tumor
Vertebral aneurysm
Platybasia
Syphilitic meningitis

NOTE: The shaded area represents the cavitation also.

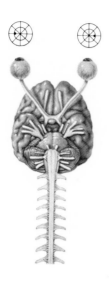

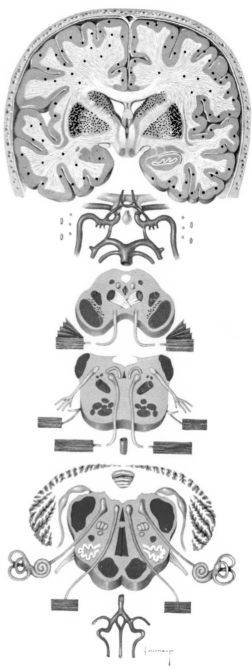

Wilson's Disease

A 16-year-old white male developed an increasing tremor and beating movements of the arms during the 3 months prior to his admission to the hospital. The family said that he had unusual outbursts of laughter and occasional difficulty swallowing food.

Neurologic examination revealed clownish faces, dysarthric speech, tremor, rigidity and rhythmic choreiform movements of both upper extremities. A Kayser-Fleischer ring was found in the limbus of the cornea on slit-lamp examination.

Treatable Diseases To Be Ruled Out
Phenothiazine toxicity
Paralysis agitans

105

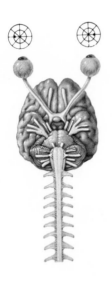

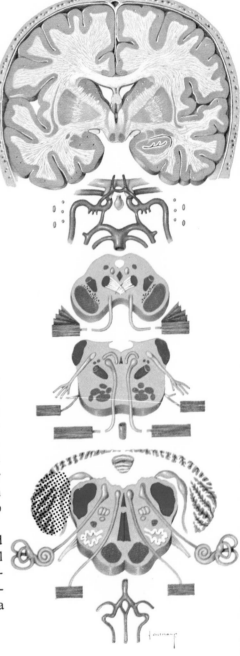

Cerebellar Abscess

A 12-year-old white girl developed a temperature of 103°, severe pain in the right ear and a mild, yellowish aural discharge 1 week prior to admission to the hospital. A diagnosis of otitis media was made, and she was treated by her local physician. One day prior to admission the temperature recurred and was associated with a severe right suboccipital headache. Her mother noted that she staggered to the right on walking. These symptoms persisted up to the time of admission.

Neurologic examination revealed horizontal nystagmus on right lateral gaze, head tilt to the right, dysdiadochokinesia and dyssynergia of the right upper extremity and a wide-based ataxia with falling toward the right.

Treatable Diseases To Be Ruled Out
Cerebellopontine angle tumor
Cerebellar tumors
Dilantin toxicity
Meningitis

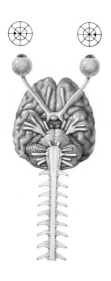

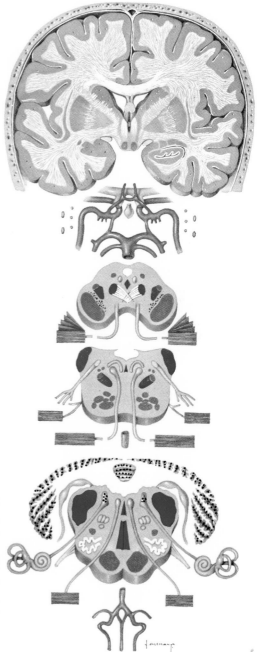

Dilantin Toxicity

A 23-year-old Negro housewife, an epileptic of several years' duration, complained of staggering while walking.

Examination revealed horizontal and vertical nystagmus, mild dysdiadochokinesia and dyssynergia bilaterally, and a wide-based ataxic gait not greatly exaggerated by closing her eyes.

Treatable Diseases To Be Ruled Out

Bromide intoxication

Space-taking lesions of the cerebellum

NOTE: Areas possibly vulnerable to Dilantin intoxication are speckled.

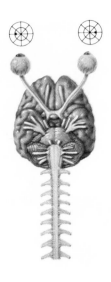

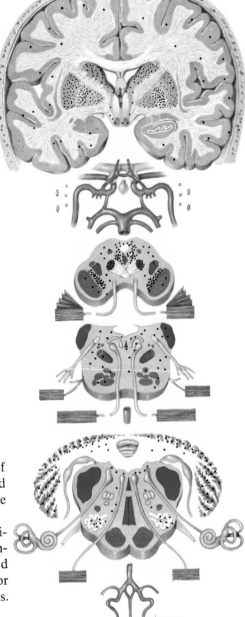

Encephalitis Lethargica

A 49-year-old white male, victim of the encephalitis epidemic of 1918, had been treated for slowly progressive parkinsonism for the past 20 years.

Neurologic examination revealed dilated areflexic pupils, paralysis of convergence, masklike faces, generalized rigidity and a coarse rhythmic tremor of the eyes, the tongue and the hands.

Treatable Diseases To Be Ruled Out
Phenothiazine intoxication
Wilson's disease
Paralysis agitans
NOTE: The brain stem is involved most severely.

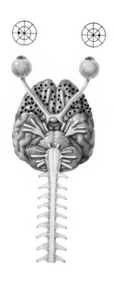

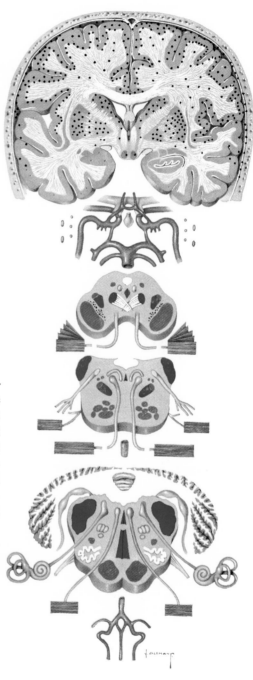

General Paresis

A 45-year-old Negro male complained of paroxysmal attacks of severe biparietal headaches for the past 2 months. His wife stated that he had been extremely forgetful and very short tempered in the past year, and had become messy with his clothes. He had been treated for a genital ulcer 13 years before, when he had received several injections.

Neurologic examination revealed inability to recall Presidents or recent events, inability to interpret proverbial phrases, disorganized affect and small irregular pupils that did not respond to light but reacted to accommodation.

Treatable Diseases To Be Ruled Out

Bromide intoxication

Lead encephalopathy

Space-taking lesions of the cerebrum

NOTE: The meninges are speckled, as they also are involved.

109

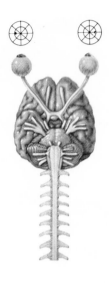

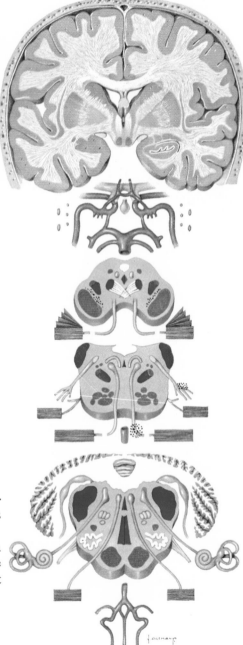

Gradenigo's Syndrome
(Petrositis)

An 11-year-old Negro boy complained of severe burning pain in his left eye.

Examination revealed a yellowish discharge from his left ear, loss of the left corneal reflex and paresis of left lateral gaze.

Treatable Diseases To Be Ruled Out

Syphilitic meningitis

Tuberculous meningitis

Cerebellopontine angle tumor

Cholesteatoma

NOTE: The nerves compressed by the lesion are speckled.

110

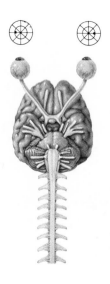

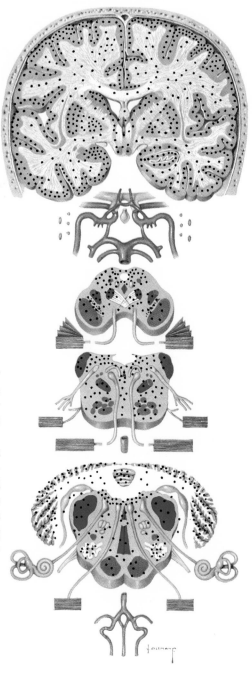

St. Louis Encephalitis

A 23-year-old Negro male developed a severe occipital headache, nausea and vomiting, and became extremely drowsy just before admission to the hospital.

Neurologic examination revealed a semistuporous male who was uncontrollable and irrational, and moved all 4 extremities freely, but there were bilateral Babinski signs. Temperature on admission was 102°. That evening he lapsed into coma and never regained consciousness.

Treatable Diseases To Be Ruled Out

Barbiturate intoxication
Diabetic coma
Insulin shock
Lead encephalopathy
Meningitis
Space-taking lesions of the cerebrum
Ruptured intracranial aneurysms

NOTE: The brain is diffusely involved.

111

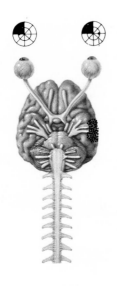

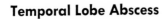

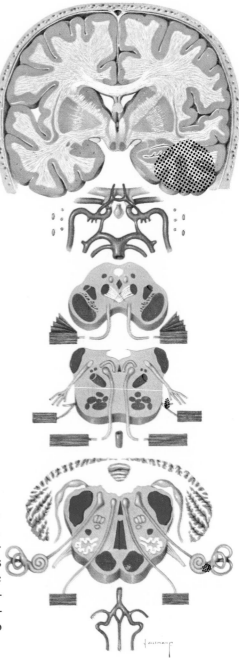

Temporal Lobe Abscess

A 28-year-old white female, who had several ear infections as a child, developed a mild, yellowish discharge from the left ear 2 weeks prior to admission to the hospital. One week prior to admission she noticed sagging of the left side of her mouth and impairment of hearing on the left. On the day prior to admission she developed a shaking chill, and the discharge increased.

Examination revealed a temperature of 101°, an early bilateral papilledema, a right homonymous superior quadranopsia, a left peripheral facial paresis and the Weber test lateralized to the right. Of particular note, she hallucinated frequently. A ventriculogram revealed shifting of the entire system to the right.

Treatable Diseases To Be Ruled Out
Other space-taking lesions of temporal lobe
Meningitis

112

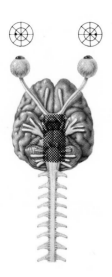

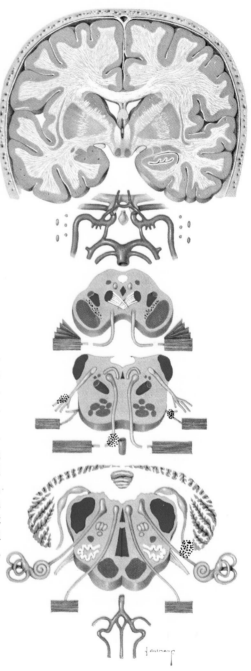

Tuberculous Meningitis

A 28-year-old white male complained of severe suboccipital headache and double vision. For the past 6 weeks he had had intermittent chills and fever, and frequent night sweats.

Neurologic examination revealed bilateral papilledema, paresis of right lateral gaze, diminished right corneal reflex, weakness in closing the left eye, and a lag of the left nasolabial fold on smiling, perceptive deafness on the left and marked nuchal rigidity. The spinal fluid revealed 850 lymphocytes per cu. mm.

Treatable Diseases To Be Ruled Out
  Bacterial meningitis
  Cryptococcal meningitis
  Syphilitic meningitis
  Wernicke's encephalopathy
  Petrositis

NOTE: Thickened meninges are represented on the longitudinal view; nerves compressed by the thickened meninges are speckled in the transverse view.

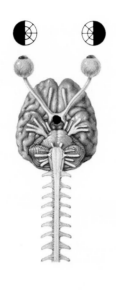

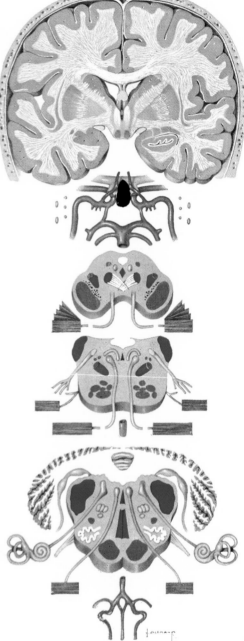

Chromophobe Adenoma

A 45-year-old white female complained of failing vision in both eyes for the past 2 years that was not improved by several different pairs of glasses. During the past 6 months she felt "like a horse with blinders on."

Neurologic examination revealed temporal pallor of both disks, bitemporal hemianopsia, and loss of axillary and pubic hair. A roentgenogram of the skull revealed a ballooned-out sella turcica.

Treatable Diseases To Be Ruled Out

Syphilitic meningitis
Craniopharyngioma
Tuberculum sellae meningioma
Aneurysms of the circle of Willis

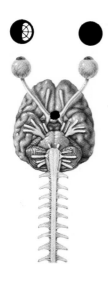

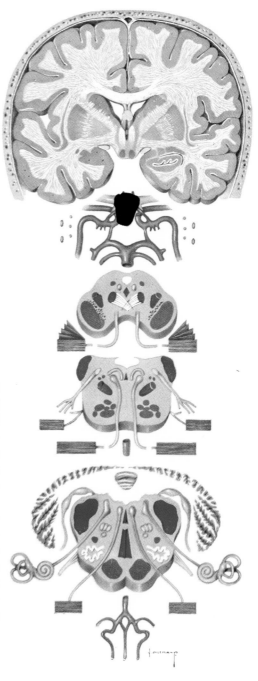

Chromophobe Adenoma

A 64-year-old Negro male had had
progressive dimming and blurring of
the vision in both eyes in the past 5
years. For the past year he had had fre-
quency of urination and excessive
thirst. One day prior to admission to
the hospital he suddenly became almost totally blind.

Neurologic examination revealed bilateral optic atrophy, inability to per-
ceive light in the left eye and a temporal hemianopic field defect on the
right. The left pupil reacted to light
only on consensual stimulation. A 24-
hour urine 17-ketosteroid excretion
was 2.8 mg.

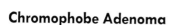

Treatable Diseases To Be Ruled Out
  Syphilitic meningitis
  Craniopharyngioma
  Tuberculum sellae meningioma
  Aneurysms of the circle of Willis

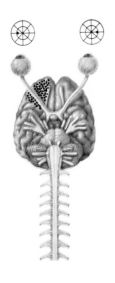

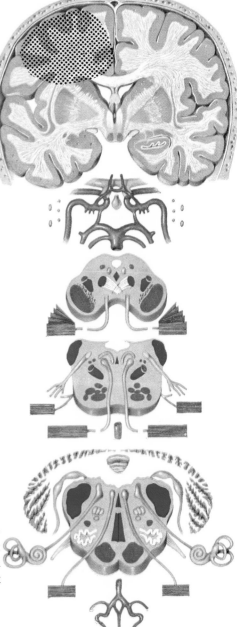

Glioblastoma Multiforme of the Frontal Lobe

A 46-year-old white male had visited his physician 1 week prior to admission to the hospital because of forgetfulness, thick speech and right frontal headaches. One hour before admission he had become semistuporous and muttered incomprehensibly.

Examination revealed facial asymmetry with straightening of the left nasolabial fold, a left hemiparesis, and a grasp and after-grasp reflex of the left hand.

Treatable Diseases To Be Ruled Out

General paresis

Bromide intoxication

Other space-taking lesions of the cerebrum

NOTE: The involved area is speckled to indicate that the tumor is infiltrative.

118

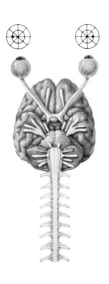

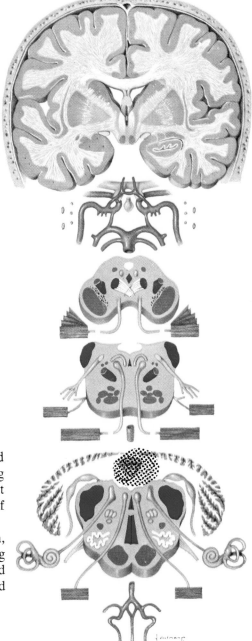

Medulloblastoma

A 9-year-old white boy had had double vision, headache and staggering gait for the past 2 weeks. For the past month he had experienced episodes of morning vomiting.

Examination revealed papilledema, bilateral paresis of lateral gaze, tilting of the head to the left and a wide-based trunk ataxia. A ventriculogram revealed dilated lateral and third ventricles.

Treatable Diseases To Be Ruled Out
Dilantin toxicity
Cerebellar abscess
Cysticercosis of 4th ventricle
Tuberculous meningitis

NOTE: The area involved is speckled to indicate that the tumor is infiltrative.

119

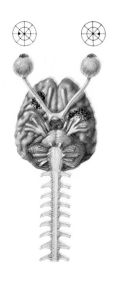

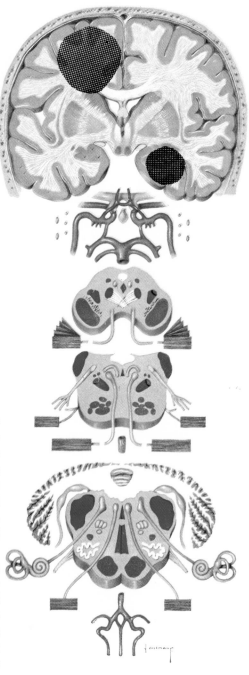

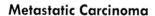

Metastatic Carcinoma

A 56-year-old white male had a sudden jacksonian convulsion that began in the left leg. He was admitted to the hospital in a stuporous state. His wife stated that he had been a heavy smoker for many years and suffered from a chronic cigarette cough. Occasionally, during the past month, he had coughed up small amounts of blood.

Neurologic examination revealed a flaccid paralysis of the left leg, questionable weakness in the left arm and a left Babinski sign. Examination the following morning revealed impairment of judgment and loss of memory for recent events in addition to the above findings.

Treatable Diseases To Be Ruled Out

Space-taking lesions of the cerebrum

120

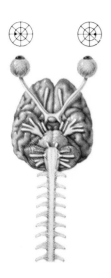

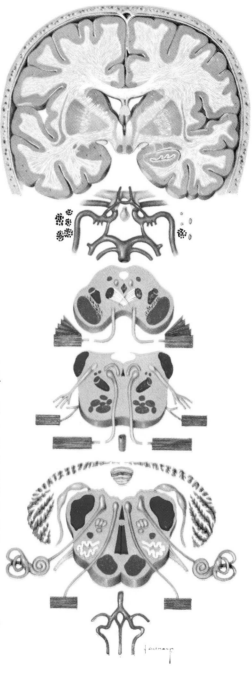

Nasopharyngeal Neoplasm (Intracranial Extension)

A 38-year-old white female complained of diplopia and right orbital and maxillary pain.

Neurologic examination revealed partial ptosis on the right, partial paralysis of gaze in all directions on the right and paralysis of lateral gaze on the left. There was no corneal reflex on the right, and there was diminished sensation to pinprick over the right cheek and forehead. Roentgenograms of the sinuses and nasopharyngoscopy confirmed the diagnosis.

Treatable Diseases To Be Ruled Out
Syphilitic meningitis
Tuberculous meningitis
Chordoma
Sphenoid ridge meningioma
Aneurysms of the circle of Willis
Cavernous sinus thrombosis
Myasthenia gravis

NOTE: The nerves that are compressed by the tumor are speckled.

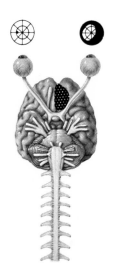

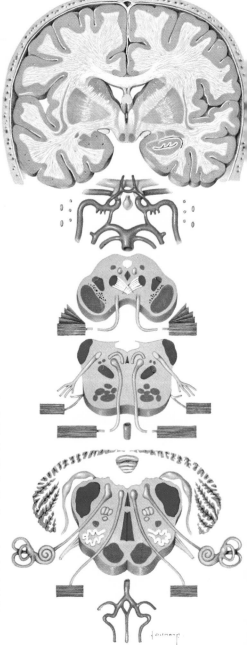

Olfactory Groove Meningioma

A 52-year-old white male complained of unrelenting frontal headache of 1 year's duration. His family noted that he had evinced very little interest in his business in the past year and that he had responded with very little emotion to the sudden death of his wife 6 months prior to his admission to the hospital.

Neurologic examination revealed left-sided anosmia, optic atrophy and concentric narrowing of the left visual field; there was papilledema of the right disk. There was considerable loss of memory for recent events.

Treatable Diseases To Be Ruled Out
General paresis
Space-taking lesions of the frontal lobe
Bromide intoxication.

122

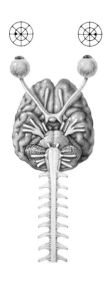

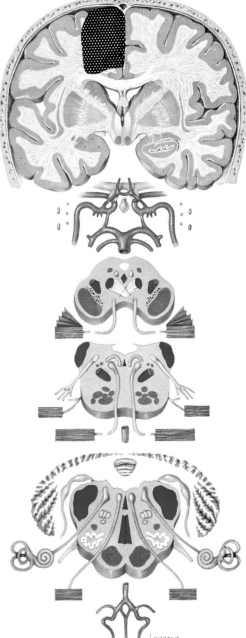

Parasagittal Meningioma

A 39-year-old white female had a 3-year history of left-sided jacksonian convulsions beginning in the left leg. One year prior to admission to the hospital she developed weakness in the left leg and intermittent right frontal headache that became progressive.

Neurologic examination revealed marked weakness of extension and flexion of the left foot and toes, hyperactive reflexes on the left side and a left Babinski sign.

Treatable Diseases To Be Ruled Out
Parasagittal abscess
Superior sagittal sinus thrombosis
Arteriovenous anomaly
Subdural hematoma

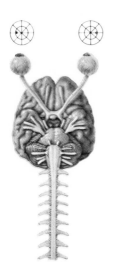

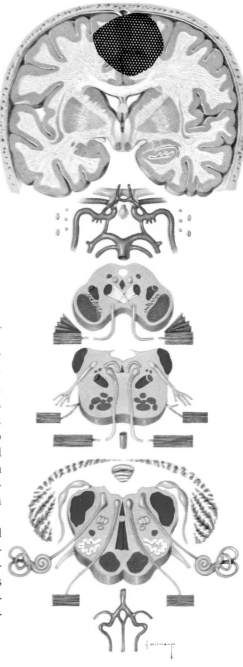

Parasagittal Meningioma

A 46-year-old Negro male had for the past 6 months experienced intermittent psychotic episodes during which he was incontinent of urine and feces and required hospitalization for 1 to 2 weeks at a time. Two months prior to admission to the hospital he had noted difficulty in walking, especially in climbing stairs. This became progressively worse. On the day of admission he had a generalized convulsion.

Neurologic examination revealed weakness, spasticity, hyperactive reflexes, Babinski signs in both lower extremities and a spastic gait. There was disorganization of thought, and the patient made many silly wisecracks during the examination.

Treatable Diseases To Be Ruled Out

Parasagittal abscess
Superior sagittal sinus thrombosis
Arteriovenous anomaly
Subdural hematoma

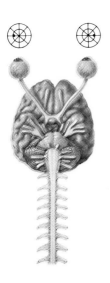

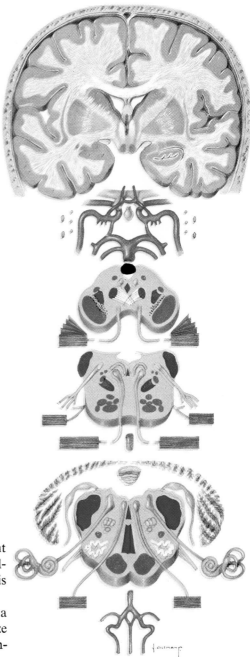

Pinealoma

A 7-year-old white boy was brought for examination because he had developed pubic hair and an enlarged penis during the past 4 months.

Neurologic examination revealed a bilateral paralysis of upward gaze (Parinaud's syndrome) and questionable paresis of convergence.

Treatable Diseases To Be Ruled Out

Wernicke's encephalopathy
Myasthenia gravis

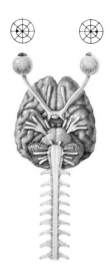

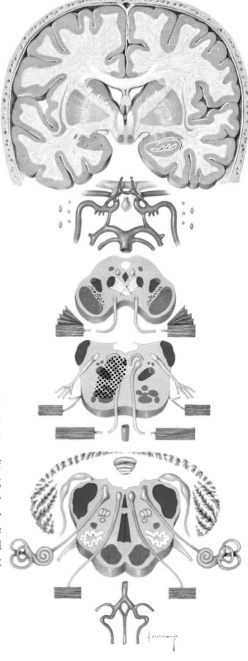

Pontine Glioma (Early)

An 18-year-old white boy complained of gradually increasing double vision for the past month. One week prior to admission to the hospital the right side of his mouth seemed to sag, and occasionally he drooled.

Examination revealed a paralysis of right lateral gaze, weakness in closing the right eyelid, a shallow right nasolabial fold and lagging of the right corner of the mouth on smiling. There were hyperactive reflexes and reduced vibratory and position sense in the left extremities.

Treatable Diseases To Be Ruled Out
Syphilitic meningitis
Tuberculous meningitis
Chordoma
Cerebellopontine angle tumor
Vertebral-basilar insufficiency

NOTE: The area involved is speckled to indicate that the tumor in infiltrative.

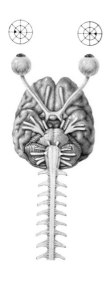

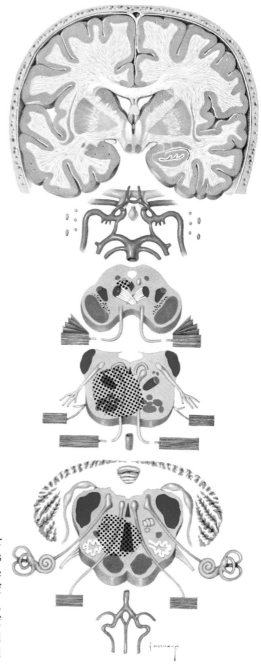

Pontine Glioma (Late)

On re-examination 3 months later there were, in addition to the previous findings, paralysis of left lateral gaze with a convergent squint, paralysis of upward and medial gaze on the right, weakness, atrophy and fasciculations of the tongue bilaterally, bilateral Babinski signs, profound loss of vibratory and position sense in all 4 extremities, and reduced sensation to pain and temperature over the right side of the face and the left trunk and extremities.

127

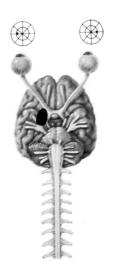

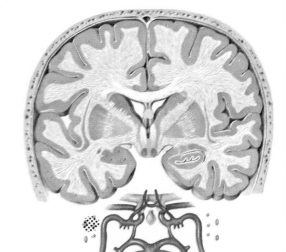

Sphenoid Ridge Meningioma

A 39-year-old Negro female complained of right frontal headache for the past 3 years. Eight months prior to admission to the hospital her husband noted that her right eye seemed to protrude. Three months prior to admission she began to complain of double vision on looking to the left.

Neurologic examination revealed right exophthalmos, papilledema of the right disk, partial paralysis of right upward, downward and medial gaze, a dilated right pupil that reacted sluggishly to light and accommodation, and a diminished right corneal reflex. A skull roentgenogram showed increased density of the right orbit and the lesser wing of the sphenoid bone.

Treatable Diseases To Be Ruled Out

Orbital cellulitis
Cavernous sinus thrombosis
Frontal lobe tumors
Aneurysms of the circle of Willis
Hyperthyroidism
Myasthenia gravis

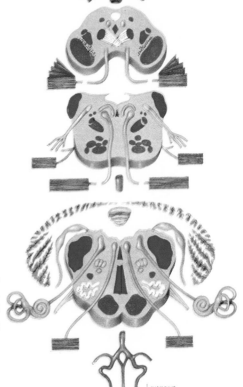

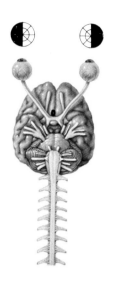

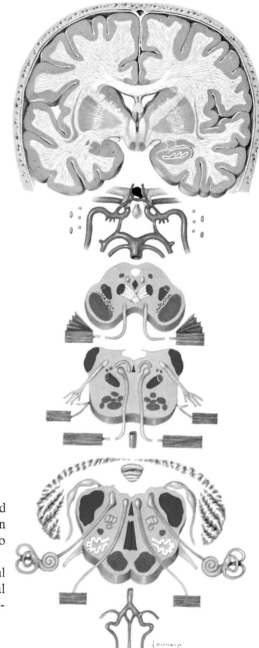

Anterior Cerebral Aneurysm

A 38-year-old white male complained of sudden onset of blurred vision in both eyes 2 days prior to admission to the hospital.

Examination revealed a bitemporal hemanopsia and questionable temporal pallor of both disks. A carotid arteriogram confirmed the diagnosis.

Treatable Diseases To Be Ruled Out
Syphilitic meningitis
Craniopharyngioma
Pituitary adenoma
Tuberculum sellae meningioma

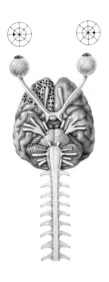

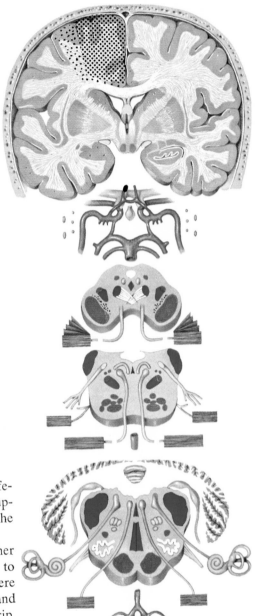

Anterior Cerebral Artery Thrombosis

A 59-year-old left-handed Negro female suddenly became unable to support her weight on the left leg, and she stumbled and fell.

Neurologic examination revealed her to be confused and disoriented and to have disorganized speech. There were flaccid paralysis of the left leg and minimal weakness of the left-hand grip. There was a left Babinski sign.

Treatable Diseases To Be Ruled Out
Space-taking lesions of the frontal lobe

Embolic encephalitis

Carotid artery thrombosis

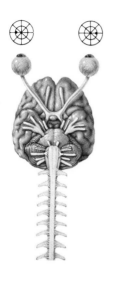

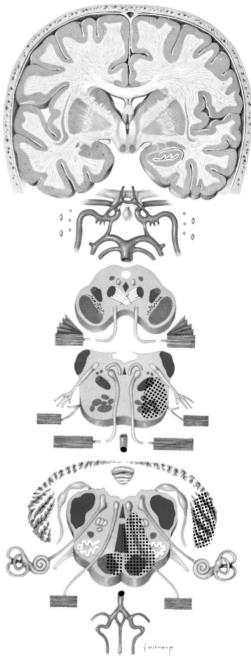

Basilar Artery Thrombosis

A 62-year-old diabetic female was admitted to the hospital with a sudden onset of slurred speech, weakness in both legs and difficulty in walking.

Neurologic examination revealed a left peripheral facial palsy, protrusion of the tongue to the left on extension, hypesthesia and hypalgesia of the right side of the body, dysmetria, dyssynergia and intention tremor of the left upper extremity, weakness of all 4 extremities but more marked in the lower extremities, and bilateral Babinski signs.

Treatable Diseases To Be Ruled Out
Vertebral-basilar insufficiency
Vertebral aneurysm

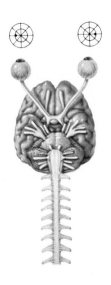

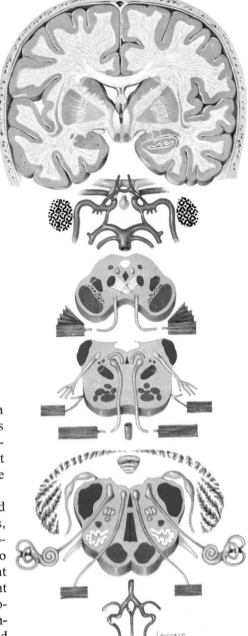

Cavernous Sinus Thrombosis

A 38-year-old Negro female, with a long history of recurrent abscesses involving the right side of the nose, developed a sudden temperature, right frontal headache and swelling of the right eye.

Neurologic examination revealed periorbital edema, chemosis, ptosis, exophthalmos and complete ophthalmoplegia on the right. There were also loss of the corneal reflex on the right and venous congestion of the right fundus. Despite antibiotics and chemotherapy, the condition progressed to involve the left eye, and the patient died 2 days later.

Treatable Diseases To Be Ruled Out
Wernicke's encephalopathy
Aneurysm of the circle of Willis

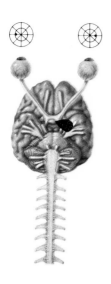

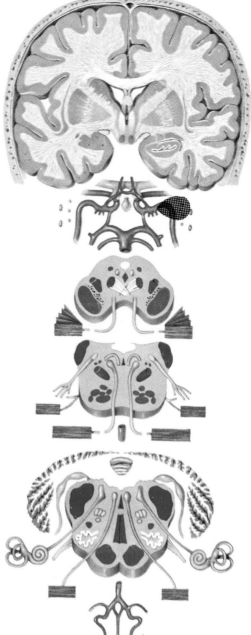

Internal Carotid Aneurysm

A 45-year-old Negro housewife noted a sudden sharp, throbbing, severe pain over the left eyebrow 1 day prior to admission to the hospital. One hour later she was unable to open her left eye.

Examination revealed a left ptosis, paralysis of upward, downward and medial gaze, a dilated areflexic pupil and loss of the left corneal reflex. A left carotid arteriogram confirmed the diagnosis.

Treatable Diseases To Be Ruled Out
Syphilitic meningitis
Tuberculous meningitis
Orbital cellulitis
Wernicke's encephalopathy
Cavernous sinus thrombosis
Sphenoid ridge meningioma
Myasthenia gravis

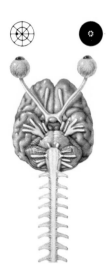

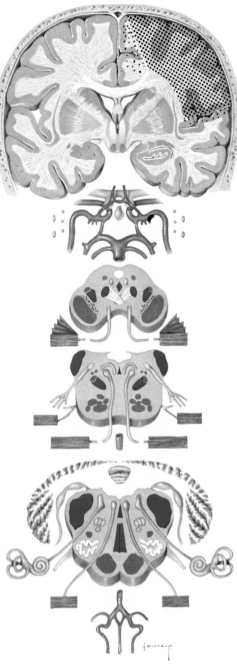

Internal Carotid Artery Thrombosis

A 69-year-old Negro male complained of intermittent episodes of right-sided weakness, lasting 15 minutes to 6 hours, for the past 6 months. One day prior to admission to the hospital he had a gradual clouding of the vision in his left eye over a period of 4 hours. That evening the right-sided weakness recurred and persisted to admission.

Neurologic examination revealed a pale left fundus, attenuation of the left retinal arteries, a cherry red spot on the left macula and a visual acuity of 20/200 o.s. There was a concentric narrowing of the left visual field. In addition, there were a right lower facial weakness and a right hemiparesis. Ophthalmodynamometric readings were 110/55 o.d. and 75/45 o.s.

Treatable Diseases To Be Ruled Out
Space-taking lesions of cerebrum
Aneurysms of circle of Willis
Common carotid thrombosis

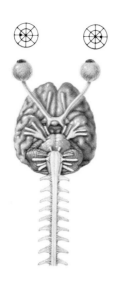

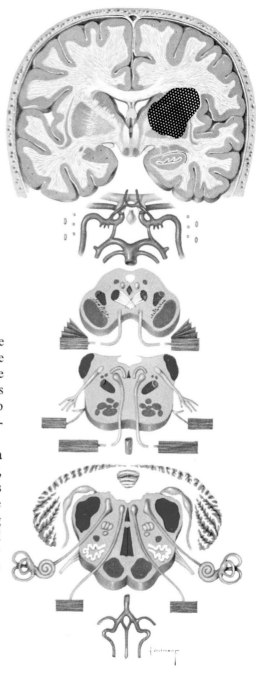

Intracerebral Hemorrhage

A 49-year-old hypertensive male had a severe bifrontal headache as he was returning home from work one evening. His wife noted that he was confused and that he went straight to bed. One half hour later she was unable to rouse him.

Neurologic examination revealed a comatosed patient, breathing deeply, with dilated, fixed pupils. There was very little spontaneous movement of the extremities, but the right arm and leg failed to move even on supra-orbital pressure. The spinal fluid was grossly bloody and under a pressure of 480 mm.

Treatable Diseases To Be Ruled Out
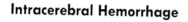
Ruptured intracranial aneurysms
Embolic encephalitis
Arteriovenous anomalies
Blood dyscrasias
Barbiturate intoxication
Diabetic coma
Meningitis

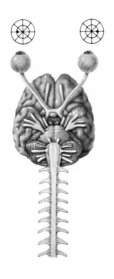

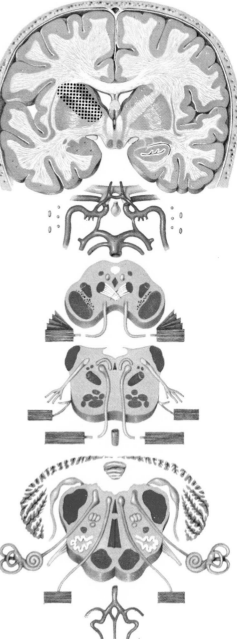

Lenticulostriatal Artery Thrombosis

A 73-year-old white female was admitted to the hospital in a semistupor and on examination was found to have a left central facial palsy, deviation of the tongue to the left, profound flaccid paralysis of the left arm and leg, and a left Babinski sign.

Treatable Diseases To Be Ruled Out

Subdural hematoma
Cerebral abscess
Ruptured middle cerebral aneurysm
Carotid artery thrombosis

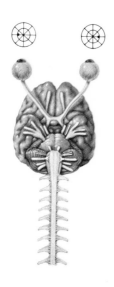

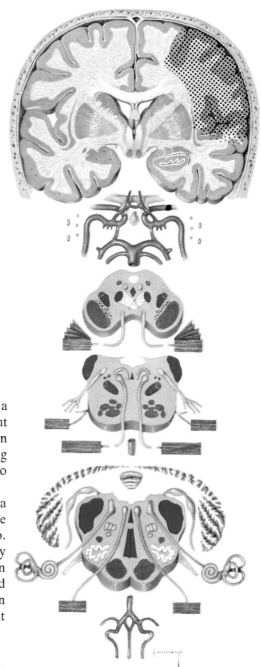

Middle Cerebral Artery Thrombosis

A 62-year-old white male noted a mild biparietal headache and slight weakness in his right arm and hand on retiring one evening. The following morning his wife found him unable to speak and his right side paralyzed.

Neurologic examination revealed a verbal aphasia, but the patient was able to understand and signify yes and no. There were a right central facial palsy and a right hemiparesis more marked in the arm than the leg. There were mild loss of position and vibratory sense on the right and astereognosis in the right hand.

Treatable Diseases To Be Ruled Out

Space-taking lesions of the frontal
and the parietal lobes
Internal carotid artery thrombosis
Embolic encephalitis

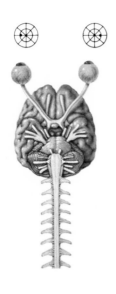

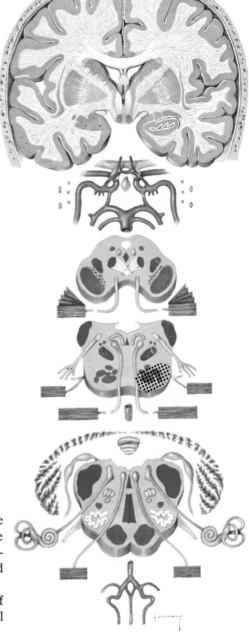

Millard-Gubler Syndrome

A 68-year-old diabetic male awoke one morning to find that he was unable to close his left eye. He also noted sagging of the left corner of his mouth and weakness in the right arm and leg.

Examination revealed impairment of left lateral gaze, left peripheral facial palsy and right hemiparesis.

Treatable Diseases To Be Ruled Out
Syphilitic vascular disease
Vertebral-basilar insufficiency

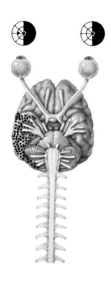

Posterior Cerebral Artery Embolism

A 28-year-old white female with a known history of rheumatic valvulitis and auricular fibrillation experienced sudden blindness in the left half of her visual field and severe occipital headache.

Neurologic examination revealed a left homonymous hemianopsia with slight macular sparing.

Treatable Diseases To Be Ruled Out
  Space-taking lesions of cerebrum
  Embolic encephalitis
  Space-taking lesions of the occipital
    or the temporal lobes
  Arteriovenous anomalies
  Vertebral-basilar insufficiency

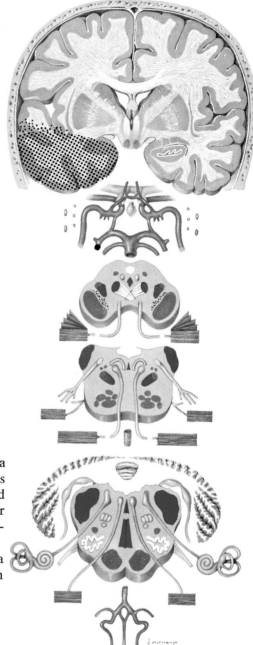

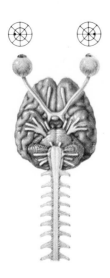

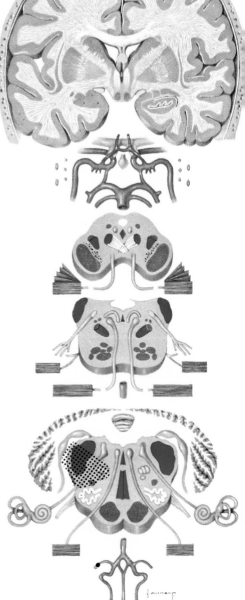

Postero-inferior Cerebellar Artery Thrombosis

A 58-year-old businessman developed suddenly a high-pitched ringing in the right ear, dizziness and right facial pain.

Neurologic examination revealed nystagmus on right lateral gaze, partial ptosis of the right eye, constriction of the right pupil, right perceptive deafness, intention tremor on finger-to-nose and heel-to-knee test on the right, loss of pain and temperature over the right side of the face and the left trunk and extremities, and falling to the right in the Romberg position.

Treatable Diseases To Be Ruled Out
Cerebellar abscess
Cerebellopontine angle tumor
Vertebral aneurysm
Vertebral basilar insufficiency
Ménière's disease

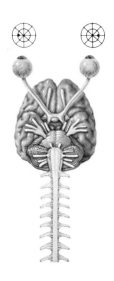

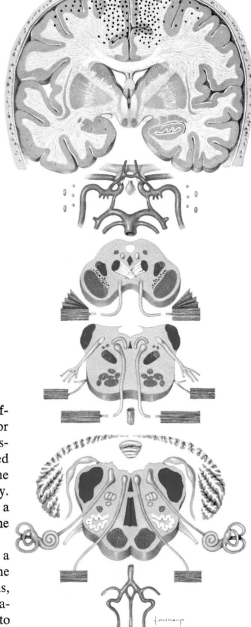

Superior Sagittal Sinus
Thrombosis

A 38-year-old Negro male had suffered from a severe postnasal drip for
several years. Two days prior to admission to the hospital the drip increased
and became yellowish in color, and the
patient complained of feeling chilly.
On the evening of admission he had a
generalized convulsion and became
stuporous.

Neurologic examination revealed a
temperature of 102°, edema of the
scalp and distention of the scalp veins,
bilateral papilledema and bilateral Babinski signs. The patient responded to
commands but was unable to speak
clearly.

Treatable Diseases To Be Ruled Out
Space-taking lesions of cerebrum

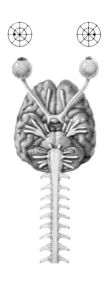

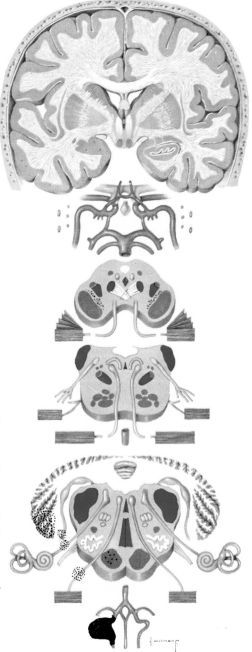

Vertebral Aneurysm

A 59-year-old white male complained of dizzy spells, staggering gait and intermittent weakness in the left hand during the past 8 months.

Examination revealed right perceptive deafness, atrophy and fasciculations of the right side of the tongue, dyssynergia of the right upper extremity, and a wide-based ataxic gait. A vertebral arteriogram confirmed the diagnosis.

Treatable Diseases To Be Ruled Out

Space-taking lesions of the cerebellum
Cerebellopontine angle tumor
Foramen magnum tumor
Vertebral-basilar insufficiency
Platybasia
Ménière's disease

NOTE: The nerves compressed by the aneurysm are speckled.

142

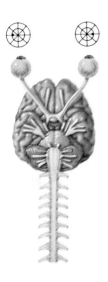

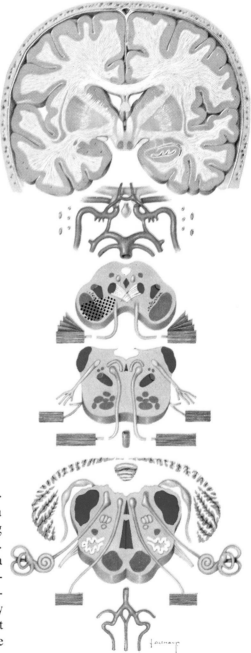

Weber's Syndrome

A 54-year-old white female complained of the sudden onset of diplopia and weakness in the left arm and leg 2 days after undergoing a hysterectomy.

Neurologic examination revealed a partial right ptosis, paresis of right upward, downward and medial gaze, a dilated right pupil that responded poorly to light and accommodation, and left hemiparesis. The intensity and the rate of cardiac rhythm were irregular.

Treatable Diseases To Be Ruled Out

Syphilitic vascular disease
Aneurysms of the circle of Willis

143

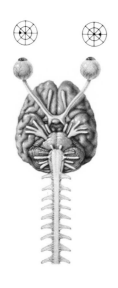

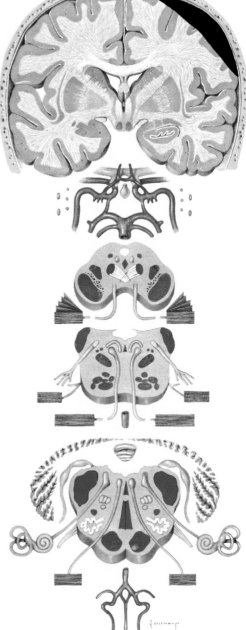

Chronic Subdural Hematoma

A 28-year-old Negro male complained of constant bifrontal headache and blurred vision of 3 weeks' duration. He had had mild intermittent frontal headaches for the past 8 months and had become irritable and difficult to live with. For the past month he had been extremely drowsy at times and would sleep 30 hours at a time. He had fallen from a moving vehicle and lacerated his scalp approximately 10 months before.

Neurologic examination revealed bilateral early papilledema, dilated left pupil and a right hemiparesis.

Treatable Diseases To Be Ruled Out

General paresis
Bromide intoxication
Subdural hygroma
Other space-taking lesions of the cerebrum

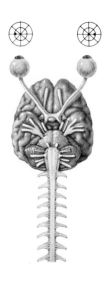

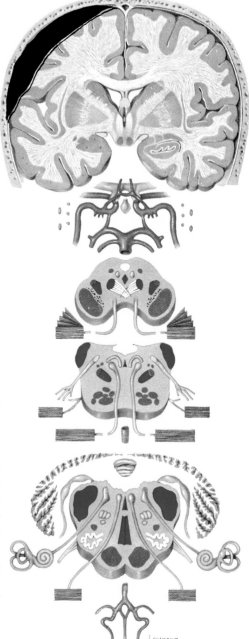

Epidural Hematoma

A 33-year-old white male sustained a severe blow on the head in an automobile accident and was brought to the accident ward in a semiconscious state. Shortly afterward it was possible to rouse him. A skull roentgenogram revealed a linear fracture of the right temporal bone. Shortly after his admission to the hospital for observation he became unconscious.

Neurologic examination revealed a blood pressure of 170/60, pulse 58, a dilated areflexic right pupil and hypoactive reflexes of the left extremities.

Treatable Diseases To Be Ruled Out
Acute subdural hematoma
Intracerebral hematoma
Depressed skull fracture

NOTE: The black line delineates the depressed dura.

145

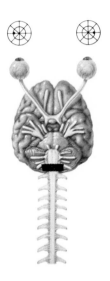

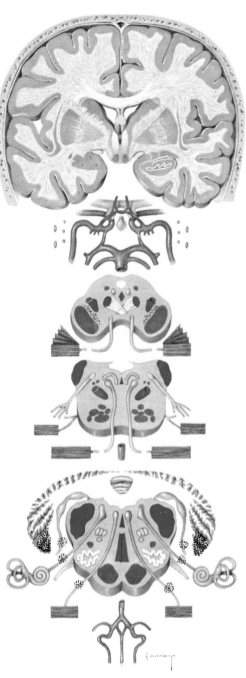

Platybasia

A 22-year-old white male complained of suboccipital discomfort, bilateral tinnitus and staggering gait intermittently for the past year.

Neurologic examination revealed loss of hearing bilaterally with a normal ratio of BC:AC, horizontal nystagmus, atrophy and fasciculations of the tongue, bilateral dysmetria, dyssynergia and intention tremor in both upper extremities, and a wide-based ataxic gait. A skull roentgenogram revealed that the atlas was occipitalized.

Treatable Diseases To Be Ruled Out
Syphilitic meningitis
Tuberculous meningitis
Cerebellopontine angle tumor
Foramen magnum tumor
Vertebral aneurysm
Vertebral-basilar insufficiency

NOTE: The solid strip on longitudinal view represents basilar impression; compressed areas are speckled on transverse views.

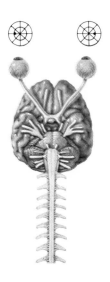

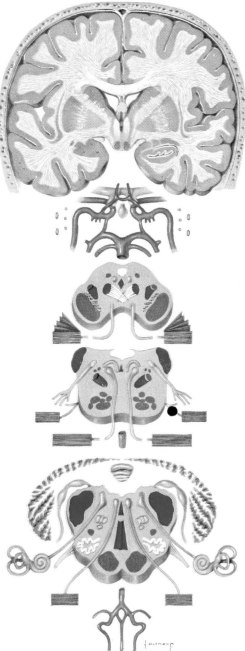

Bell's Palsy

A 27-year-old Negro female awoke one morning with numbness of the left side of her face, excessive tearing from the left eye and thick speech.

Examination revealed inability to close the left eye, Bell's phenomenon, straightening of the left nasolabial fold and inability to retract the left side of the mouth on smiling or grimacing.

Treatable Diseases To Be Ruled Out
Petrositis
Syphilitic meningitis
Cholesteatoma
Cerebellopontine angle tumor
NOTE: The area of pathology is spotted.

147

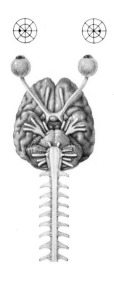

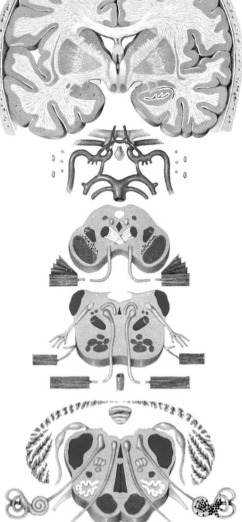

Ménière's Disease

A 45-year-old white male had had episodes of vertigo, tinnitis and fullness in his left ear lasting 2 to 6 hours at a time for the past 3 years. More recently he had had loss of hearing in his left ear that was especially noticeable during the attacks.

Neurologic examination during an attack revealed nystagmus on left lateral gaze, left perceptive deafness, especially to low tones, and unsteadiness in the Romberg position.

Treatable Diseases To Be Ruled Out

Syphilitic meningitis
Petrositis
Cerebellopontine angle tumor
Cholesteatoma
Vertebral aneurysm
Vertebral-basilar insufficiency

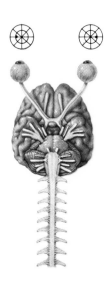

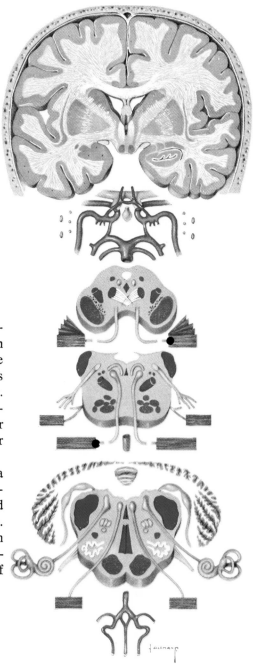

Myasthenia Gravis

A 26-year-old white female complained of intermittent double vision that occurred more often toward the end of the day. Several different pairs of glasses resulted in no improvement. One week prior to admission to the hospital the patient had had an upper respiratory infection, and 2 days later she developed ptosis of the left eye.

Neurologic examination revealed a left ptosis, partial paralysis of left upward, medial and downward gaze, and total paralysis of right lateral gaze. There was complete remission of both symptoms and signs after the intravenous administration of 0.5 ml. of Tensilon.

Treatable Diseases To Be Ruled Out
    Syphilitic meningitis
    Tuberculous meningitis
    Wernicke's encephalopathy
    Sphenoid ridge meningioma
    Aneurysms of the circle of Willis
NOTE: The affected myoneural junctions are
    spotted.

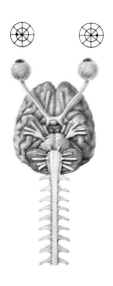

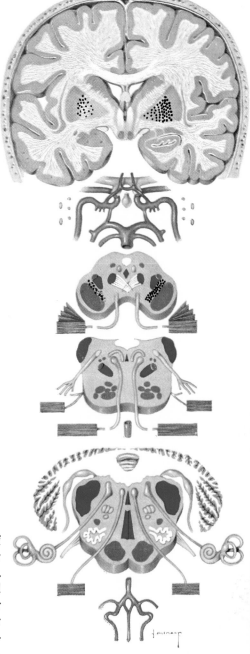

Paralysis Agitans

A 50-year-old nurse complained of difficulty in writing plainly and tremor in her right hand of 2 month's duration.

Neurologic examination revealed masked faces, mild involuntary tremor at rest in the right hand and, to a lesser extent, in the left hand, and short-stepped gait with a semiflexed posture.

Treatable Diseases To Be Ruled Out
Wilson's disease
Phenothiazine intoxication

Appendix A

Parts of examination listed according to tract, nucleus, region or system examined

Cerebrum

Orientation in time, space and person
Attention span
Memory
Ability to interpret proverbial phrases
Affect
Ability to follow simple or complex commands
Ability to differentiate right from left
Serial sevens
Arithmetic
Spelling
Reading
Writing
Feeding
Speech (perceptive, nominal, syntactic, expressive aphasias)
Two-point sensibility, vibratory and position sense
Stereognosis
Muscle power
Sucking and grasp reflexes
Visual fields
Reflexes

Extrapyramidal System

Facial expression
Check for Myerson's eye signs
Affect
Speech (monotonous)
Muscle tone
Check for spontaneous movements (choreiform, athetoid)
Gait and station
Propulsion, retropulsion test
Check for Kayser-Fleischer ring

Cerebellar System

Nystagmus (horizontal, rotary)
Speech tests ("Round, rugged rock," "Methodist-Episcopal," etc.)
Finger-to-nose test (look for intention tremor)
Supination-pronation test
Patting test
Rebound test
Ability to button clothes
Heel-to-knee test
Gait and station
Babinski-Weil test
Ability to circle chair clockwise and counterclockwise
Leg-swinging test of Wartenberg
Muscle tone (hypotonia)
Physiologic reflexes

Vestibular System

Check for:
  Dissociated nystagmus
Disconjugate deviation of eyes
Vertical nystagmus

151

Cranial Nerves

I
   Olfactory sense (vanilla, mint, spice)

II
   Funduscopic examination
   Visual fields
   Visual acuity
   Check for:
      Exophthalmos
      Enophthalmos

III, IV, VI
   Pupillary light, accommodation and consensual reflexes
   Extraocular movements
   Palpebral fissures
   Red-glass test

V
   Corneal reflex
   Jaw reflex
   Bite
   Sensation of face
   Trigger zones for neuralgia

VII
   Ability to close the eyes tightly
   Ability to wrinkle the forehead
   Ability to whistle
   Ability to show the teeth
   Taste on anterior two thirds of the tongue
   Orbicularis oculi reflex

VIII
   Otoscopic examination
   Wrist-watch test
   Weber's and Rinne's tests
   Audiogram
   Caloric tests
   Check for:
      Nystagmus
      Past-pointing
      Romberg

IX
   Pharyngeal sensation
   Taste (posterior one third of tongue)
   Gag reflex

X
   Palate and uvula position and movements
   Ability to say A, E, I, O, U
   Ability to swallow
   Gag reflex

XI
   Ability to turn head from side to side
   Ability to shrug the shoulders
   Sternocleidomastoid bulk and tone

XII
   Ability to protrude the tongue
   Bulk of tongue
   Check for:
      Tremors
      Fasciculations

Pyramidal Tracts

Tests of muscle power:
  Hand grip
  Adduction and abduction of fingers
  Extension of hand
  Flexion and extension of forearm and arm
  Abduction of arm
  Flexion and extension of thigh
  Flexion and extension of lower leg
  Flexion and extension of foot and toes
Physiologic reflexes:
  Pectoralis
  Biceps
  Triceps
  Brachioradialis
  Digitorum
  Superficial abdominal

  Cremasteric
  Patellar
  Achilles

Pathologic reflexes:
  Palm to chin
  Hoffmann
  Trömner
  Babinski
  Oppenheim
  Gordon
  Chaddock
  Rossolimo
  Marie-Foix
  Patellar and ankle clonus (pathologic accentuation of physiologic reflexes)
Muscle bulk and tone (spasticity)
Rectal tone and control
Bladder tone and control

Posterior Column and Medial Lemniscus

Vibratory sense
Position sense
Finger-to-nose test (eyes closed)
Graphesthesia

Stereognosis
Two-point sensibility
Gait and station
Check for Romberg

Spinothalamic Tracts and Ventral Commissure

Pain
Superficial touch

Hot-cold test
Test for sacral sparing

Sensory Root

Superficial pain
Deep pain
Touch
Vibratory and position sense
Straight-leg-raising test
Palpate sacrosciatic notches
Deep sensation of testicles and Achilles tendon

Physiologic reflexes (as listed under Pyramidal Tracts)
Muscle tone
Gait
Check for trophic changes
Bladder and rectal tone and control

Motor Horn or Root

Tests of muscle power (as listed under Pyramidal Tracts)

Physiologic reflexes (as listed under Pyramidal Tracts)

Muscle bulk and tone (measure with tap)

Bladder and rectal tone and control

Check for fasciculations

Myoneural Junction

Tests of muscle power

Ability to count, chew and blink eyes without fatiguing

Muscle

Tests of muscle power

Muscle bulk

Myotonic reflex (Delayed relaxation of hand grip)

Gait

Peripheral Nerve

Test for all sensory modalities (as listed under Sensory Root)

Muscle power

Physiologic reflexes

Muscle bulk and tone

Check for:

Trophic and vasomotor changes

Nerve and muscle tenderness

Skull

Sutures and fontanelles

Shape

Size

Check for bruits and exostosis

Neck

Check for:

Nuchal rigidity

Kernig's sign

Brudzinski's sign

Diminished carotid pulsations

Lhermitte's sign

Brun's syndrome

Massage carotid sinus

Occlude one carotid at a time

Skin

Check for:

Vasomotor changes

Hyperhidrosis or anhidrosis

Redness

Temperature changes

Trophic changes (ulcers, nail deformities)

Angiomas

Fibromas

Congenital anomalies (cleft lip, etc.)

Café-au-lait spots

Bones and Joints

Check for: Charcot's joint
    Kyphosis   Pes cavus
    Scoliosis   Hammer toe

Autonomic System

Pulse   Palpebral fissures
Blood pressure   Sweat function
Intestinal motility   Mecholyl test
Pupils   Cocaine test

Endocrine System

Temperature   Nails:
Pulse   Shape
Blood pressure   Thickness
Skin: Tongue:
    Texture   Size
    Thickness   Coating
    Pigmentation   Color
    Temperature   Breasts:
    Dermatologic disorders   Size
Hair: Clitoris:
    Texture   Size
    Distribution   Check special eye signs:
Subcutaneous tissue   von Graefe's sign
Fat: Joffroy's sign
    Distribution   Möbius' sign
    Amount   Patellar and Achilles reflexes (sus-
Bones: tained)
    Shape   Check for:
    Size   Trousseau's sign
Teeth: Chvostek's sign
    Shape
    Thickness

Appendix B

Signs characteristic of involvement of one tract, nucleus or region

Sign	Tract, Nucleus or Region Involved
Pathologic reflexes (Babinski, etc.)	Pyramidal tract
Hyperactive reflexes	Pyramidal tract (not pathognomonic unless unilateral)
Spastic gait	Pyramidal tract
Spastic neurogenic bladder	Pyramidal tract
Grasp reflex	Premotor cortex (frontal lobe)
Fasciculations	Anterior horn
Bitemporal hemianopsia	Optic chiasma
Astereognosis	Parietal lobe
Vertical nystagmus	Brain stem
Involuntary tremor at rest	Extrapyramidal system

Signs characteristic of involvement anywhere along a pathway or system of two or more tracts, nuclei or regions (from peripheral to central)

Loss of power	Muscle Myoneural junction Peripheral nerve Anterior horn or root Pyramidal tract Frontal lobe
Muscle atrophy	Muscle Peripheral nerve Anterior horn or root
Anesthesia	Peripheral nerve Sensory root Posterior column Medial lemniscus Ventral commissure Ventral spinothalamic tract Thalamus Parietal lobe
Analgesia	Peripheral nerve Sensory root Ventral commissure Lateral spinothalamic tract Thalamus

Loss of vibratory and/or position sense	Peripheral nerve Sensory root Posterior column Medial lemniscus Thalamus Parietal lobe
Romberg	Sensory root Posterior column Medial lemniscus
Nystagmus (excluding ocular nystagmus)	Labyrinth Vestibular nerve Vestibular nuclei Medial longitudinal fasciculus Flocculonodular portion of cerebellum

Appendix C

Group 1: The signs in the extremities are exclusively motor

Below the Foramen Magnum

Disease	Tract, Nucleus or Region Involved
Amyotrophic lateral sclerosis	Anterior horn and pyramidal tract
Lead neuropathy	Anterior root and motor portion of peripheral nerve
Muscular dystrophy and myotonia dystrophica	Muscle
Myasthenia gravis	Myoneural junction
Poliomyelitis	Anterior horn
Progressive muscular atrophy	Anterior horn

Above the Foramen Magnum

Space-taking lesions	Frontal lobe
Anterior cerebral artery occlusions	Frontal lobe
Lenticulostriatal artery occlusion or hemorrhage	Internal capsule
Middle cerebral artery occlusion	Motor strip of frontal lobe
Parkinsonism	Globus pallidus substantia nigra
Primary cerebellar atrophy	Cerebellum

Group 2: The signs in the extremities are exclusively sensory

Below the Foramen Magnum

Arsenical neuritis	Primarily sensory portion of peripheral nerve
Herpes zoster	Sensory root
Intramedullary tumor (early)	Ventral commissure
Space-taking lesions of the cord (early)	Sensory root
Syringomyelia	Ventral commissure
Tabes dorsalis	Sensory root, posterior column

Group 3: The signs in the extremities are combined sensory and motor diseases: all others

References for Further Reading

1. Alpers, B. J.: Clinical Neurology, Philadelphia, Davis, 1954.
2. Blackwood, W.: Atlas of Neuropathology, Baltimore, Williams & Wilkins, 1949.
3. Davidoff, L., and Feiring, E.: Practical Neurology, New York, Landsberger Medical Books, Inc., 1955.
4. DeJong, R.: The Neurological Examination, New York, Hoeber, 1958.
5. Forster, F.: Modern Therapy in Neurology, St. Louis, Mosby, 1957.
6. Haymaker, W.: Bing's Local Diagnosis in Neurological Diseases, St. Louis, Mosby, 1956.
7. Holmes, G.: Introduction to Clinical Neurology, Edinburgh, Livingstone, 1952.
8. Merritt, H. H.: A Textbook of Neurology, Philadelphia, Lea & Febiger, 1955.
9. Purves-Stewart, J.: The Diagnosis of Nervous Diseases, London, Arnold, 1931.
10. Steegmann, A. T.: Examination of the Nervous System, Chicago, Year Book Pub., 1956.
11. Walshe, F.: Diseases of the Nervous System, Baltimore, Williams & Wilkins, 1958.

Glossary

Adie's syndrome. Tonic pupil together with absence of the patellar reflex.

altitudinopsia. A defect of the upper or the lower half of the visual field.

ankle clonus. A series of rhythmic hyperactive ankle jerks produced by forcible and brisk dorsiflexion of the foot.

apraxia. Inability to perform purposeful motions.

astasia-abasia. Apparent inability to walk or stand due to some mental conflict.

astereognosis. Inability to recognize objects by the sense of touch.

ataxia. In-co-ordination of muscular action.

athetosis. Recurrent, slow and continual change in position of the fingers and the toes or any part of the body.

Babinski sign. Extension of the great toe with fanning of the other toes on exciting the sole.

Babinski-Weil test. A test to determine vestibular and cerebellar function, performed by having the patient walk forward and backward 10 or more times with the eyes closed. In cerebellar or vestibular disease the patient deviates to the side of the lesion.

Benedikt's syndrome. Contralateral hemianesthesia and involuntary choreiform movements and homolateral oculomotor paresis in occlusion of the paramedian basilar branch supplying the red nucleus and the medial lemniscus.

Brudzinski's sign. A sign of meningeal irritation in which raising the recumbent patient's head causes involuntary flexion of the thighs.

Brun's syndrome. A form of episodic vertigo, headache, disturbance of vision and feeling of blacking out on flexion or extension of the head, seen in posterior fossa tumors.

café-au-lait spots. Areas on the skin of a "coffee with cream" color often associated with von Recklinghausen's disease.

caloric test. A test for vestibular function, performed by placing water at various temperatures in the external auditory meatus and observing for nystagmus.

Chaddock's sign. Extension of the great toe and fanning of the other toes on stroking the lateral malleolus and the dorsum of the 5th metatarsal.

Charcot's joints. Joint enlargement with osteoarthritis due to trophic disturbances in patients with tabes dorsalis, syringomyelia, etc.

chorea. Irregular and involuntary action of the muscles of the extremities and the face.

Chvostek's sign. A sign for tetany in which tapping the face in front of the ear produces spasm of the facial muscles.

disconjugate deviation of eyes. Gaze palsy more severe at the medial rectus than at the lateral rectus, or vice versa.

dissociated nystagmus. Nystagmus in which the movements of the two eyes are dissimilar.

dysarthria. Imperfect pronunciation of words or phrases causing them to be slurred together.

dysdiadochokinesia. Difficulty in performing rapid alternating movement.

dysmetria. Disturbance of ability to measure distance and orientation in space while performing acts (especially with the eyes closed).

dyssynergia. Loss of co-ordination in the performance of skilled or un-skilled movements of the arms and the legs.

fasciculations. An in-co-ordinate contraction of skeletal muscle in which groups of muscle fibers innervated by the same neuron contract to-gether.

fibrillations. A local quivering of denervated muscle fibers usually not de-tectable by gross examination.

Foster Kennedy syndrome. Descending atrophy of one disk with papilledema of the other.

Foville's syndrome. Abducens palsy, plus homolateral facial palsy, plus homolateral gaze palsy.

Gordon's sign. Plantar extension of the great toe when the calf muscles are squeezed firmly.

graphesthesia. Ability to recognize numbers written on the skin.

grasp reflex. Automatic clenching of fist when an object is placed in the hand.

hammer toe. Condition of the second toe in which the proximal phalanx is extended extremely while the two distal phalanges are flexed.

Hoffmann's sign. A test for overactive tendon reflexes in which the tapping of the nail of the index or the middle finger causes flexion of the thumb.

Hoover's sign. A sign to differentiate true hemiplegia and hysterical hemi-plegia. In true hemiplegia the patient thrusts the normal leg down-ward on attempting to raise the paralyzed leg. In hysterical hemiplegia the patient attempts to raise the paralyzed leg without thrusting the normal leg downward.

hysteria. A psychoneurotic disorder, characterized by extreme emotionalism involving disturbances of the psychic, the somatic and the visceral function.

internuclear ophthalmoplegia. Gaze palsy, more severe at the medial rectus than at the lateral rectus, or vice versa.

Kernig's sign. Inability fully to extend the leg when the thigh is flexed. A sign of meningeal irritation.
kyphosis. Angular curvature of the spine, the convexity of the curvature being posterior.

Lasègue's sign. Extreme sensitivity to stretching the sciatic nerve trunk on straight-leg-raising.
Lhermitte's sign. A sensation of an electric shock shooting into the extremities on flexion of the neck, occurring most typically in multiple sclerosis.

Marie-Foix sign. Forced dorsiflexion of toes and withdrawal of leg on transverse pressure of the tarsus.
Millard-Gubler syndrome. Abducens palsy, plus homolateral "peripheral" facial palsy, plus crossed hemiplegia.
Minor's sign. A method of rising to the standing position seen in patients with sciatica in which the weight is supported on the healthy side and the affected leg is bent, one hand being placed on the back.
Myerson's eye signs. Uncontrollable blinking of the eyes when an object is brought near them or the brow is tapped.
myotonic reflex. Sustained tonic contraction of a muscle on reflex stimulation, seen in myotonia dystrophica.

nucleus. A group of neuron cell bodies in the central nervous system concerned with a particular function.
nystagmus. An oscillatory movement of the eyeballs.

Oppenheim's sign. Plantar extension of the great toe in response to firm stroking of the medial border of the tibia from above downward.

palm-to-chin reflex. Contraction of the homolateral mentalis muscle on stroking the palm, indicating pyramidal tract disease.
Parinaud's syndrome. Paralysis of vertical gaze, plus disturbance of convergence due to a lesion in the peri-aqueductal gray of the mid-brain.
past-pointing. On attempting to bring the finger to a desired point the finger either falls short or passes beyond to the right or the left of the point.
pes cavus. A form of club foot in which the arch is high.
platybasia. A developmental deformity of the occipital bone and the upper cervical spine in which the foramen magnum is small and misshapen, the atlas is occipitalized, and the axis impinges on the brain stem.

propulsion. A falling forward in walking, observed in paralysis agitans, in which the patient cannot stop at will.

quadranopsia. Hemianopic defect delimited by the horizontal meridian.

reaction of degeneration. No reaction of the muscle to faradic current and diminished response to a galvanic current.

red-glass test. A test for subclinical forms of diplopia, performed by placing a red glass before one eye, thus producing a false image before that eye. The patient with diplopia will see two images.

retropulsion. A running backward observed in paralysis agitans.

Rinne's test. A test to ascertain the ratio of air to bone conductivity, performed by placing a vibrating tuning fork first to the mastoid process and then just adjacent to the ear (after the subject no longer hears the fork over the mastoid process).

Romberg's sign. Swaying to one side, forward or backward, with the eyes closed while standing with the feet close together.

Rossolimo's sign. On stroking or tapping the plantar surface of the toes, plantar flexion of the toes occurs when there are lesions of the pyramidal tract.

sacral sparing. Sparing of sensory loss in the distribution of the sacral and the lower lumbar nerves in intramedullary lesions of the cord.

scoliosis. Lateral curvature of the spine.

scotoma. A dark spot in the visual field.

space-taking lesions. Lesions such as tumors, abscesses, hematomas, fractures, herniated disks, etc., that occupy space inside the skull or the spinal column that normally is occupied by the components of the central nervous system.

spasticity. An increased tonus or tension of a muscle that is associated with an exaggeration of the deep reflexes.

steppage gait. The peculiar high-stepping gait seen in tabes dorsalis and certain peripheral neuropathies.

tomography. The technic of making roentgenograms of plane sections of solid objects.

tract. A bundle of axonal fibers that perform a similar function.

Trömner's sign. With the fingers of the patient partially flexed, tapping the volar aspect of the tip of the middle and the index fingers, causing flexion of all four fingers and thumb, indicating a pyramidal tract lesion.

Trousseau's sign. A sign for tetany in which carpal spasm can be elicited by compressing the upper arm.

trunk ataxia. A disturbance of station and gait, with loss of balance and tendency to fall backward, due to in-co-ordination of trunk movements with those of the extremities.

two-point sensibility. Ability to discriminate one or two points placed at varying distances apart on the skin.

Wartenberg's leg-swinging test. With the patient in a sitting position and the legs hanging freely, pendular swinging movements of the legs can be produced by raising and suddenly releasing them.

Weber's syndrome. Paralysis of the oculomotor on the side of the lesion and the extremities and hypoglossus on the opposite side.

Weber's test. A test for lateralization of auditory impairment, performed by placing vibrating tuning fork on the vertex in the mid-line.

Wernicke's hemianopic pupillary response. Absence of pupillary reaction to light from the "blind" side in hemianopsia.

INDEX

The Numbers in boldface type refer to the color plates.

169